Liang Zhen Pu
Eight Diagram Palm

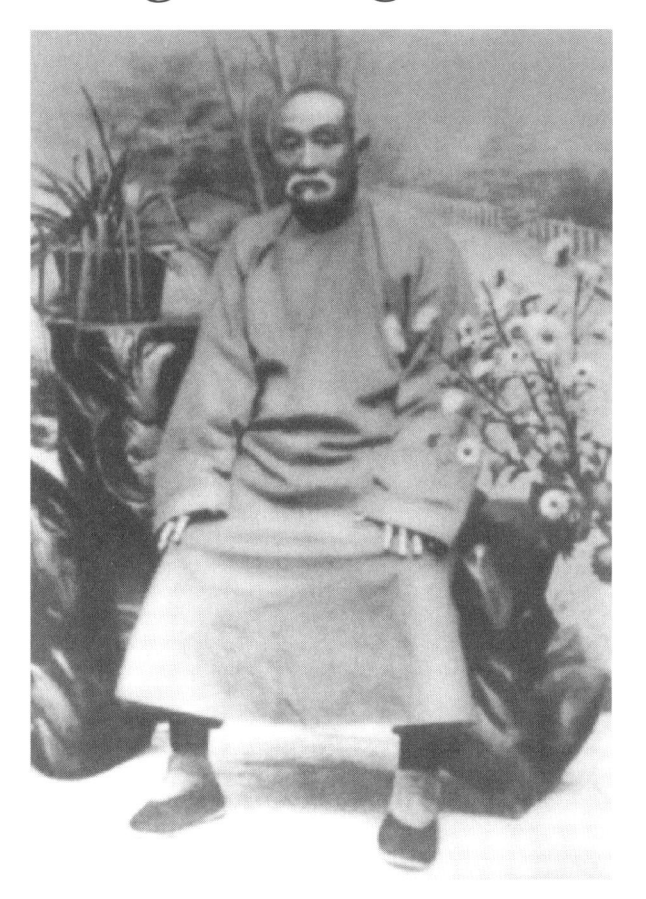

梁振蒲八挂掌

By Li Zi Ming
Translated by Huang Guo Qi
Compiled and Edited by Vincent Black

High View Publications, Pacific Grove, CA

Liang Zhen Pu Eight Diagram Palm

Copyright © 1993 Vincent Black
ISBN 1-883175-00-3
All Rights Reserved

Published by High View Publications
P.O. Box 51967
Pacific Grove, CA 93950

Photographs of Zhao Da Yuan in Chapter 6 by Dan Miller

Printed in the United States of America

The author and publisher of the book are not responsible for any injury which may result from following the instructions contained herein.

Before embarking on any of the physical activities described in this book, the reader should consult his or her physician for advice regarding their individual suitability for performing such activity.

TABLE OF CONTENTS

Editor's Acknowledgments iv
Preface v
Forward to the English Translation viii
In Memoriam x
Forward by Master Li Zi Ming xi

CHAPTER I - Introduction 1
   1. What kind of martial art is Eight Diagram Palm? 1
   2. Nomenclature of Eight Diagram Palm 2

CHAPTER II - Characteristics of Eight Diagram Palm 7
   1. Circle Walking and Footwork 7
   2. Strategy and Tactics of Out Flanking 12
   3. Exercise Method Conforms to Natural Principles 13
   4. Combination of Movement and Stillness and of Firmness and Gentleness . 15
   5. The Eight Contraries 17

CHAPTER III - Some Main Points in Practice of Eight Diagram Palm 23
   1. Careful Prevention of Three Fatal Errors 23
   2. Combination of Attack Skill and Art 24
   3. Guidelines for Practice 26

CHAPTER IV - Compilation of Theory on Eight Diagram Palm 31
   1. Sixteen-Word Formula of Eight Diagram Palm 31
   2. Formulae of Hand, Eye, Body, Method and Step 32
   3. Circle Walking Song of Eight Diagram Palm 35
   4. Song of Eight Diagram Palm Walking About the Circle 38
   5. Song of Eight Diagram Palm Applications 41
   6. Song of Eight Diagram Palm 43
   7. Method of Eight Boxings in Eight Diagram Palm 44

CHAPTER V - Formulae Handed Down From Mr. Dong Hai Chuan 47
   1. Thirty-Six Songs and Annotations 48
   2. Essential Formulae of Forty-Eight Methods and their Annotations . . . 79

CHAPTER VI - Exercises and Figures of Eight Diagram Palm 111

Editor's Postscript 153
About the Translator 154

EDITOR'S ACKNOWLEDGMENTS

First and foremost I have to give my deepest thanks to Master Li Zi Ming for his willingness to share his time, knowledge and wisdom with me. The privilege of having studied with him will always remain a high point in my life.

It is a privilege to have worked with Mr. Huang Guo Qi over the last five years in preparing *Liang Zhen Pu Eight Diagram Palm*. His patience and commitment to the task is something I will never forget. Without him this project could not have been undertaken.

I want to acknowledge my wife, Kim, for the endless hours of support in the numerous readings, rewrites and typing. Without her encouragement, the task would still be before me unfinished. And to that end, I have to acknowledge and thank my publisher, Dan Miller, for his prodding and personal energy volunteered to produce a book the quality of which is worthy of the subject.

I was honored that my senior school brother Mr. Zhao Da Yuan has graciously consented to stand for the photographs in the section presenting the Old Eight Palms (*Lao Ba Zhang*). His contribution will be appreciated by all those striving to perfect their form.

Finally, I have to express my heartfelt gratitude to my friends and colleagues, Dr. Ken Fish and Tim Cartmell, whose meticulous translational critique has afforded a greater accuracy in the translation, thus preserving fine points that no doubt would have otherwise been lost.

PREFACE

It is a great honor to have been able to work with Master Li Zi Ming to help bring his book *Liang Zhen Pu Eight Diagram Palm* to the English speaking readership. It is one of those rare and unexpected opportunities of life that seem to come from nowhere, yet on looking back, I realize that I have actually been moving toward it in many ways for some time. I can only hope to succeed in doing what justice I am capable of in rendering this work, the treatise of an eighty year old Ba Gua Zhang Grandmaster and Chinese scholar, into an appreciable format for my fellow practitioners to share.

While there have been some excellent previous publications on the art of Ba Gua Zhang that clearly presented the general theory and main points of the system, Master Li has presented an in-depth exposition of all the "internal" ramifications involved in performing and utilizing this sophisticated fighting system. Never before has a treatise by a master of such long term experience and insight been made available to those outside the Chinese community.

While on the surface this may appear as a rather straight forward process, the rendering was complicated by several serious considerations. One area that was problematic in the process was selecting the appropriate terminology and expression that would retain "all of the meanings" that Master Li would superimpose into one idea. While the pictographic nature of the Chinese written language does this as well as any, the linear flow of the structure of the English written language does not lend itself easily to such application.

Another consideration that constantly arose in the rendering was the amount of repetition in the book. While in a standard western writing it may be construed as redundant and tedious, Master Li's repetitious style is not without purpose. He is a grandmaster of Ba Gua Zhang having taught his art steadily for many decades thereby gaining profound insights and perfecting his wisdom in teaching. In observing the typical learning process, he was astute in discerning the common stumbling blocks and manners in which most practitioner err in their early training. The entire work is constantly interspersed with his admonitions and wise counsel on how to study and how to teach properly to avoid wasting time and attain the highest level of achievement possible. These remarks should be diligently noted in relation to and in conjunction with the particular points that are being presented. His repetitious expression is an effort to emphasize these points to the acolyte so that their significance will not be over looked and will hopefully lead to more rapid progress in training.

There is yet another purpose and that is to continually splice and interweave the various components and concepts, both internal and external, to produce a "wholistic" image as it were; this idea of all the different characteristics and attributes associated with the Ba Gua Zhang system coalescing into a singular natural expression speaks to the highest goals of internal boxing.

And finally, there are expressions contained in the original text that, while they may be translated literally to mean one thing, in a martial arts connotation they specifically mean something quite different. Some are commonly understood among boxers, while others arcane to all but the most elder masters. His many references to classical martial art proverbs and abstruse terms provide enriching images that are very nearly lost to contemporary practitioners. To ferret out all of these expressions from the general text is no easy task and I have no doubt made some errors. For this, I beg understanding both from Master Li and the general readership. I welcome comments and questions from all quarters in an effort to fulfill Master Li's directive of "enduring work in the company of men to unveil the real Ba Gua."

>   Vincent Black
>   Winter of 1992
>   Pembroke, Virginia

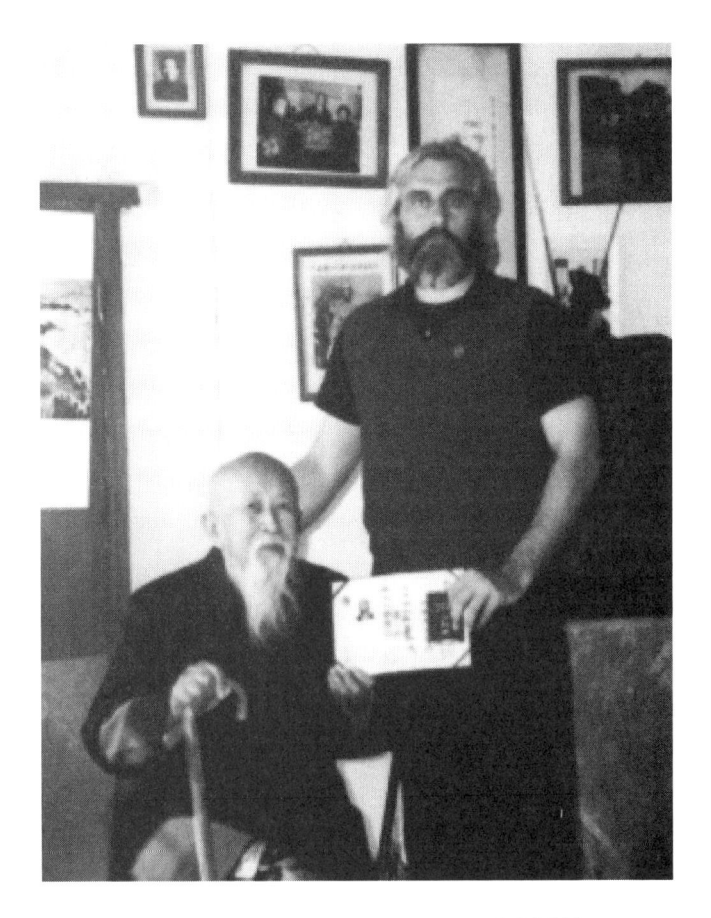

Vince Black with his teacher Li Zi Ming

FORWARD TO THE ENGLISH TRANSLATION

In 1982, on the 100th anniversary of Dong Hai Chuan's death, Li Zi Ming published this book privately in Beijing, China. Until now, this book was only available in Chinese and one could only obtain it from Li Zi Ming himself. Li had a very limited number of books printed and thus they were never offered for sale to the general public.

When I was visiting with Li Zi Ming in 1991, he gave me a copy of this book and asked if I could publish it for him in English. I told him that I would do my best. After returning to the United States, I related this story to Vince Black. Vince had studied with Li Zi Ming for two consecutive years in China and it turns out that Li had made the same request of Vince. Vince told me that he had had his translator, Huang Guo Qi, translate this book into English after his first visit with Li in 1989. When Vince went back to Beijing to study with Li in 1990, he and his translator sat with Li every morning for a month and discussed the details of each of the songs contained in the book at great length.

By spending countless hours discussing the songs and formulae which form the theoretical foundation of Eight Diagram Palm method with a Master with over 60 years experience in the art, Vince was able to gain valuable insights. While he used his experience in compiling and editing this book, his knowledge extends far beyond what is written here. The songs and formulae of Eight Diagram Palm were written by the art's founder so that initiate students could easily remember and transmit the principles of the art. As such, the songs and formulae are not designed to teach, but to help initiate students remember what they were taught.

In my capacity as the editor and publisher of the *Pa Kua Chang Journal*, I have had the opportunity to interview dozens of Eight Diagram Palm masters in China. Whenever I ask questions about the principles or fundamentals of the art, the Master being interviewed will typically begin to recite one or more of the songs. Memorization of these songs was mandatory for students in China. However, without experiential understanding of the songs through physical practice of the art, the songs do not hold as much meaning.

Through his 30 years of experience in the martial arts and his intense study with Li Zi Ming, Vince Black has gained an experiential knowledge of the principles contained within this book and is able to skillfully demonstrate that knowledge in practical application. All practitioners of the Eight Diagram Palm method will gain valuable insights through individual study of the principles contained herein. However, those who are unable to unravel any of the deep meaning contained in these songs and/or Li Zi Ming's annotation are encouraged to contact Vince Black. His work and effort in carrying on the tradition of Li Zi Ming's Eight Diagram Palm method in the United States is greatly appreciated by all practitioners of the art.

>Dan Miller
>Winter 1992
>Pacific Grove, CA

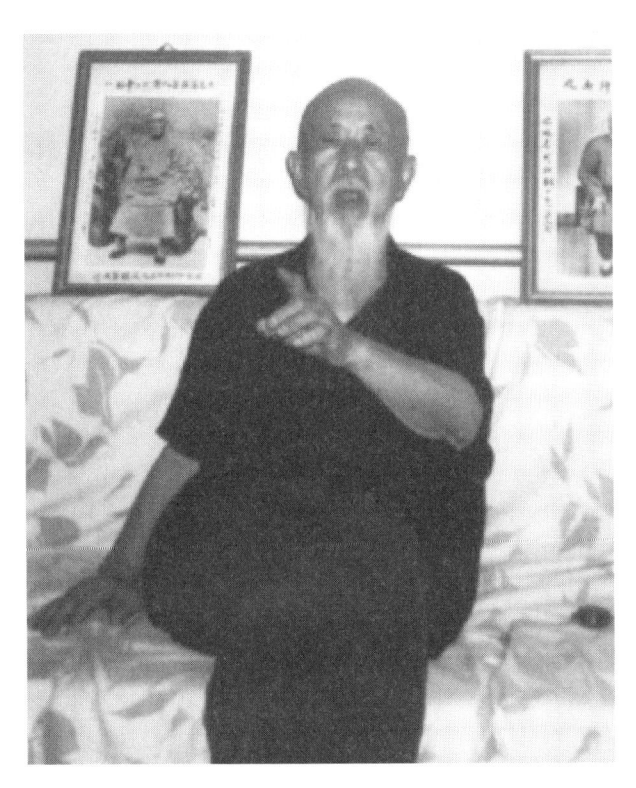

**Li Zi Ming discussing the "songs"
of Eight Diagram Palm**

IN MEMORIAM

This first English edition of *Liang Zhen Pu Eight Diagram Palm* is dedicated to the memory of Grandmaster Li Zi Ming, one of the last great Ba Gua Zhang masters of this century.

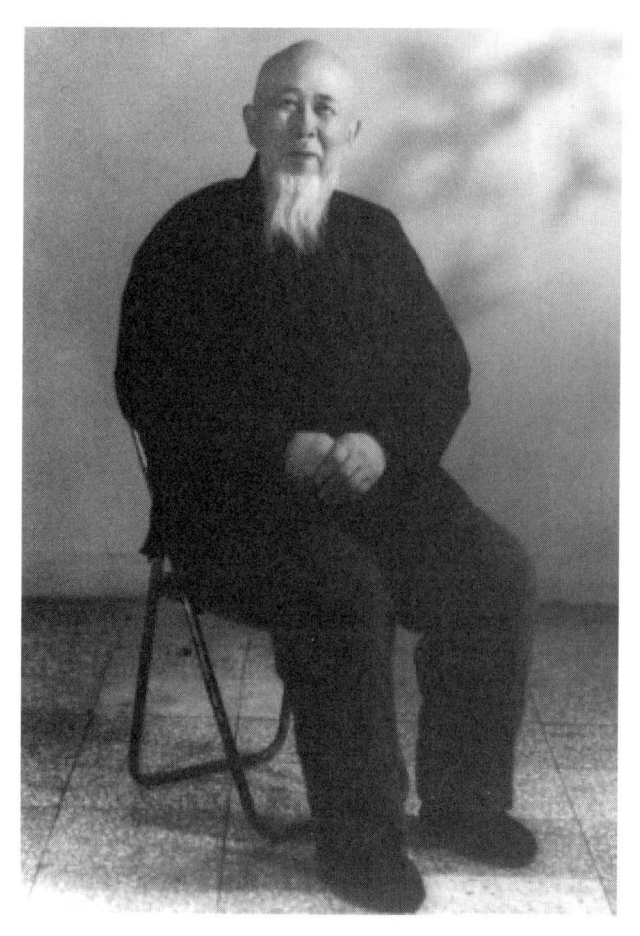

Eight Diagram Palm Master Li Zi Ming
June 24, 1900 - January 24, 1993

FORWARD

by Master Li Zi Ming

Eight Diagram Palm (*Ba Gua Zhang*), one of the internal schools of boxing (*Nei Jia Quan*) in China, is an outstanding cultural heritage. Until now, few books on the Eight Diagram Palm method have been published. Although several books were published prior to liberation, due to the passage of time and diminishing interest, there are very few copies of those presently existing. After liberation, the martial arts experienced a revitalization having been promoted as part of our national heritage with exhibition games being held regularly. With this renewed interest in martial arts, many books on this subject have also been published. But, only one major book on Eight Diagram Palm - "Eight Diagram Palm" written by Mr. Jiang Rong Qiao - has been published[1]. Presently, the popularity of Eight Diagram Palm has spread North and South of the Yangtze River with more and more enthusiasts of this boxing method. Therefore, the single treatise on Ba Gua Zhang written by Mr. Jiang seems insufficient to stand alone as the sole banner of the many Ba Gua Zhang enthusiasts and, in deed, will require subsequent contributions by those of us who long to see the limitless proliferation of this excellent martial art. To that end, I wrote and compiled *Liang Zhen Pu Eight Diagram Palm* as an overall introduction and reference for those enthusiasts, present and future, of the Eight Diagram Palm boxing method.

My aim in writing *Liang Zhen Pu Eight Diagram Palm* is to enhance the flourishing development of this martial art which, in time, I believe will strengthen the health of the people and help to vitalize China. At the same time, I wrote this book in memory of Mr. Dong Hai Chuan, the originator of the Eight Diagram Palm in Beijing, and my teacher, Mr. Liang Zhen Pu. Therefore, I wrote down the Thirty-six Words Formula and Forty-eight Methods Formula in the Eight Diagram Palm handed down from Mr. Dong Hai Chuan to my teacher, Mr. Liang Zhen Pu, and then to me. These traditional songs are the compass with which the Eight Diagram Palm practitioners measure and chart the course of their training. They are the keys to the precious essentials that make the Eight Diagram Palm the distinctive art that it is. In earlier times, because of prejudice among schools of thought and the more conservative nature with which people practiced their particular martial art, these songs would not be handed down to people so openly. Now I present all these songs and subsequent annotations for the public in order for enthusiasts to master the essentials of the Eight Diagram Palm system.

This marvelous boxing method, when practiced properly according to the essentials, can develop the practitioner's physical health to restore the essence, tonify the brain, dispel illness, prolong life and maintain optimum vitality which, in the end, will serve as a contribution for the socialist construction of a better China. To that end, I wrote down my personal experiences in sixty years of practice of the Eight Diagram Palm with full annotations in regard to both my teacher's and grand-teacher's traditional songs in order to help clarify difficult passages for the generations to follow in hopes of attracting valuable opinions and encouraging more complete works on the Eight Diagram Palm which would be written by my colleagues.

Due to the limitation of the author's knowledge, the incomplete descriptions and mistakes cannot be avoided theoretically and literarily. The author sincerely hopes that the readers would offer their valuable suggestions and criticism.

I would like to express my thanks to Mr. Fan Zhen Yuan of Wuxi Municipality, who offered his assistance and Mr. Zhang Xiu Lin of Jiujiang Municipality, who helped to write explanations for the exercise movements.

Li Zi Ming
Spring of 1982
Beijing, China

Endnotes

[1] Mr. Jiang was highly regarded as a foremost authority in Ba Gua Zhang, therefore, this publication has given him singular recognition while there may have been some minor publications by other less celebrated practitioners. Special consideration needs to be given to the understanding that in the political reformation period of the Communist Party in China there was little exchange in and out of mainland China of these kinds of materials. Consequently, there were things published by some boxers of some note, that may not have received sufficient circulation in China.

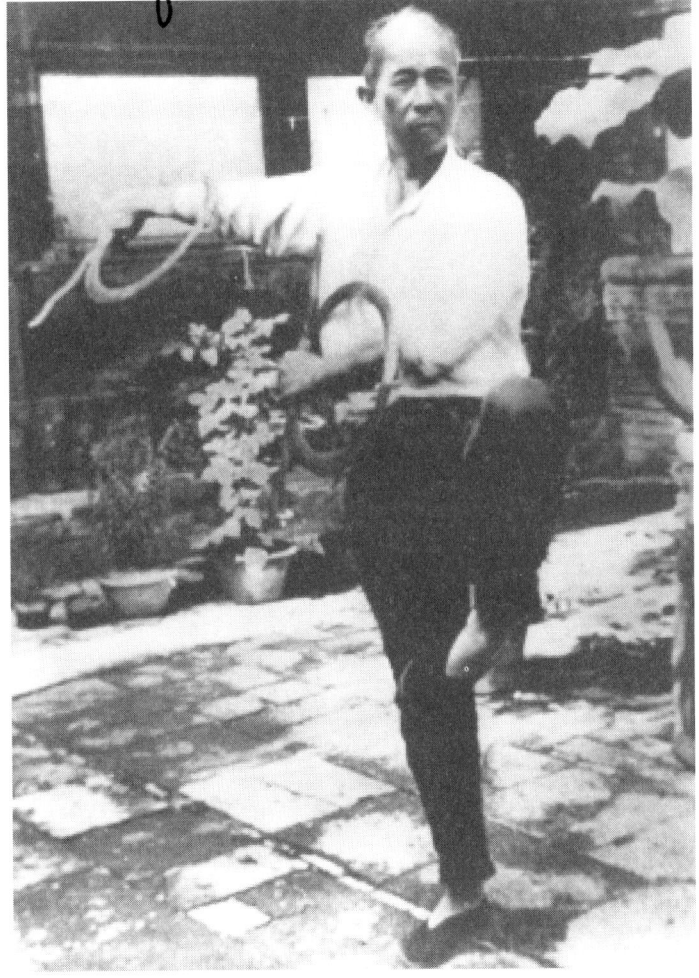

Li Zi Ming, circa 1955, practices with the Wind and Fire Rings

CHAPTER I

INTRODUCTION

1. What kind of martial art is Eight Diagram Palm?

In man's struggle with the natural world, internally with disease and externally with physical aggression, the possession of skills, and methods to develop those skills, to deal with the challenges of life has from the beginning and continues to vitally influence the development of civilization. The Chinese people created and developed martial arts and boxing skills through centuries of prolonged struggle and perseverance. Chinese martial arts rank high on the list of contributions in the cultural heritage of China. This is partly due to its importance, historically, in being applied in the defense against foreign invasions in ancient times, as well as providing an expression of physical culture that promotes good health and personal self-defense capabilities. The Chinese martial arts have a long history rich in content, diverse in schools of thought, and encompassing a wide variety of distinctive skills. However, in the general classifications there are two major divisions of martial arts: the internal schools (*Nei Jia Quan*) and the external schools (*Wai Jia Quan*).

Ba Gua Zhang, or Eight Diagram Palm, is an internal boxing system and as such has its own requirements. While in external school boxing it is primary to train the body well to perform external skills and functions both in solo practice and in working with partners, it is also necessary in internal school boxing to develop *Qi* cultivation in combination with the execution of these external skills. The proverb of the martial arts masters "exercise skin, tendons, bones externally and cultivate *Qi* internally" refers to this type of exercise, i.e., "the skill for guiding exhalation and inhalation" mentioned in the Taoist school is combined with the Chinese martial arts. By integrating *Qi Gong* principles, the martial arts can be improved to become even more profound. By the practice of the martial arts, *Qi Gong* can be promoted

1

and developed more expansively. Due to the combined internal and external training, the physical body (muscles, tendons, bones) is exercised while the vital energy[1] and strength are mutually developed. Gradually, the functions of the internal organs are enhanced and the physical constitution is thereby improved. Therefore, it is traditionally considered a good art for health and longevity.

Eight Diagram Palm is one of the most recently developed boxing methods in the history of classical Chinese martial arts[2]. It is difficult to investigate and impossible to ascertain exactly when it started and by whom it was created. However, it is known that this art was developed based on the best principles of various boxing skills and through prolonged practice and refinement by the Chinese Taoists. In the Ching Dynasty Mr. Dong Hai Chuan was the first master to accept apprentices and teach his skills in Beijing over a century ago. Although one hundred years is not much time in Chinese history or in the development of an art form, the exquisite blending of movement and stillness, firmness and gentleness, internal energy and external energy intrinsic in Eight Diagram Palm, is clearly superior to other boxing methods. It's suitability for practice by male, female, old and young alike has popularized it to the broad masses. Not only has it proliferated vigorously to the areas of the Yangtze River, but to the far reaches of the world as well. This was demonstrated when in the relocation of Mr. Dong Hai Chuan's tomb, enthusiasts from all over the world sent financial support in memory of him. This attests to the contributions in general that the Eight Diagram Palm system offers the human struggle against disease and the promotion of health and longevity.

2. Nomenclature of Eight Diagram Palm

In order to understand why this boxing method was named Eight Diagram Palm one needs to first understand the concept of the eight diagrams. The following is the configuration combining both the congenital and acquired eight diagrams:

Qian Father (pure yang), heaven (sky), strength, creativity, active, Yang, cold, head

Kan Second son, water (cloud), enveloping, dangerous, ear

Introduction

Gen Third son, mountain, stubborn, immovable, contrary, hand

Zhen First son, thunder, springtime, active, rousing, moving, foot

Xun First daughter, wind, wood, gentle, penetrating, thigh

Li Second daughter, fire, sun, lightning, clinging, eye

Kun Mother, earth (ground), yielding, receptive, passive, belly

Dui Third daughter, lake (marsh), rain, autumn, joyful, mouth

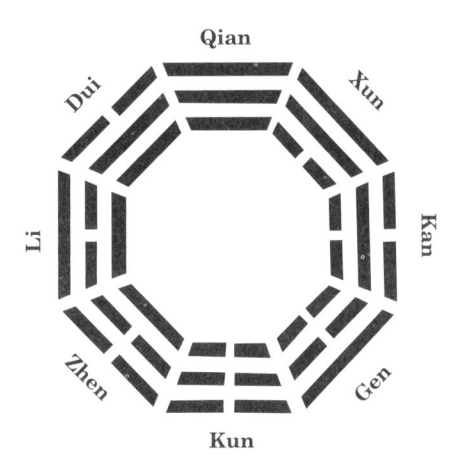

Fu Xi's Pre-Heaven Arrangement

These eight words refer to the eight fundamental diagrams in the "*Zhou Yi*" (*I-Ching*)[3]. In all there are sixty-four diagrams in the *Zhou Yi* and there are sixty-four tactics in the Eight Diagram Palm.

The Eight Diagram Palm was created and developed on the theory of the principle of change. During practice it is necessary to walk the circle in eight directions, i.e., the so-called four steps and four oblique angles. While circle walking one must keep the upper body still while moving the lower body. When releasing power, it is necessary to play gently with firmness and firmly with gentleness. "Substantial and insubstantial (weighted and unweighted, firm and supple) must all be clearly differentiated, so that the body acts as a single unit with unified force (trained strength)."

Liang Zhen Pu Eight Diagram Palm

At that time, Mr. Dong Hai Chuan taught only eight postures (i.e., Eight Great Palm (*Ba Da Zhang*) or Old Eight Palm (*Lao Ba Zhang*)) to conform to teachings and positioning of the eight diagrams. It's changes and tactics also imply several changes of the eight diagrams. In training with other practitioners or in combat, whenever the opponent changes strokes and gestures, I also change my strokes and gestures immediately to counter their position. Because energy and power are obtained from the walking and turning, continuous walking on the circle and left and right turning are basic exercises of the system. The changing of strikes and turning on a circle characterize the specific form in which Eight Diagram Palm is practiced and is usually determined by strategies and tactics of self-defense. The walking principles are congruent with the variations of the eight diagrams and their relative position within the overall theory of the *I-Ching*. This is how the name Eight Diagram Palm was derived. Because the strokes and gestures are ever changing and difficult to anticipate, whenever it is mentioned, people often say that there are sixty-four palms or three hundred and eighty-four palms. Actually, there are only eight palms and only eight signs like the eight trigrams. The reason other people say these things is that the strokes and gestures change according to the circumstances and so frequently that people are unable to cope with them.

In Eight Diagram Palm the feet walk and turn continuously like a swimming dragon, the postures change quickly like a nimble eagle (kite hawk), the strokes and gestures change swiftly and the palms strike like an active ape. The result is a visually impressive form; light but not floating, deep but not stagnant, and an excellent physical culture. It is little wonder that it has spread around the world and been accepted by so many.

Endnotes

[1] Due to the numerous and varied applications of the term "*Qi*," the editor has in some cases replaced the term "*Qi*" with "vital energy," in other cases with "breath," and in other cases left it unchanged for greater clarity in the reading.

[2] While it is typical of Chinese martial artists to lend authority to their personal method by attributing long lineage that reaches far back in history, Master Li was unique in his position that Eight Diagram

Introduction

Palm, rather than having ancient roots, characteristically developed as a culmination and refinement of the most sophisticated principles gleaned from the previous millennia of martial arts evolution.

[3]The *Zhou Yi* arrangement is an ordering of events or conditions in a manner that allows one to foretell to some degree the upcoming developments based on present and recently past developments and their interrelationship. This ancient method is structured in a matrix of symbols derived from various combinations of yin and yang in an ordered sequence and representing concepts which are simultaneously nonspecific and yet archetypical of the human condition and, as such, can be applied to all dimensions of life's situations. This foresight enables one to change in accord with present and upcoming possibilities to leave one in a position of advantage. This process reflects the importance the ancient Chinese attached to the principle of change in dealing with the myriad trials of life. For more information refer to any of a number of translations of the *I-Ching*.

Liang Zhen Pu Eight Diagram Palm

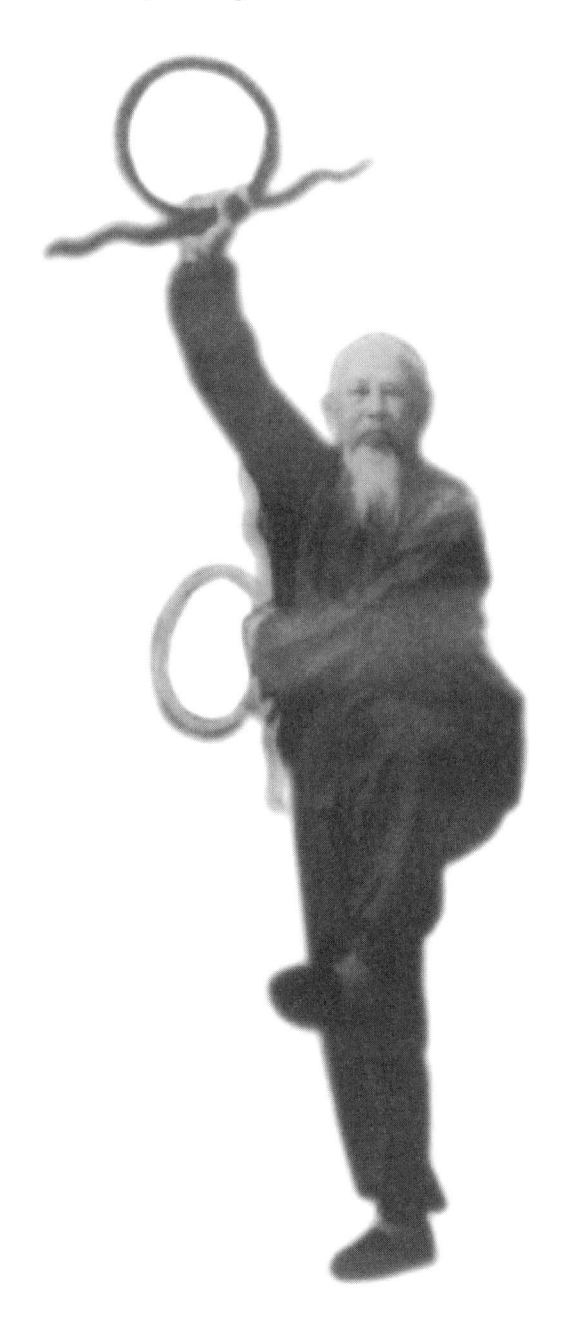

CHAPTER II

CHARACTERISTICS OF EIGHT DIAGRAM PALM

1. Circle Walking and Footwork.

The primary characteristic in Eight Diagram Palm is the circle walking. Circle walking is the major basic method in applying Eight Diagram Palm techniques and, therefore, the most important basic exercise.

Mr. Liang Zhen Pu used to say: "Circle walking in the Eight Diagram Palm is derived from and understood through comprehending principles of nature; it is obtained from the practice of the walking and turning method." Therefore, the beginner must learn walking, turning and training the legs as the basic exercises in order to realize the goal of cultivating energy. Only by sufficient training of the legs can the internal energy be well cultivated. Without leg strength there would be no internal energy. There is a proverb in Chinese martial arts: "Practicing boxing without training the legs would be a reckless venture and practicing boxing without practicing strength and skills would leave one with nothing in the end." Only by the long-term, painstaking practice of circle walking can the lower body be stable and able to step quickly, deeply and balanced.

When cultivated to the highest level of proficiency, circle walking serves to regulate physiological functions by balancing metabolism, improving the physical constitution and enhancing the overall level of health. Therefore, it is not only a way to maintain health but also a key to longevity. Furthermore, it is a good method for vanquishing enemies. In confrontation with an opponent, the mobility gained from continuous walking already puts one in an advantageous position tactically. When it's necessary to change steps in a critical moment, the legs and feet can instantly perform the very important function of mobility. With swift and various changes of the palm, one can take the offensive and execute a defense freely, all taking place within the continuous movement. The

Liang Zhen Pu Eight Diagram Palm

ability to endure in a prolonged struggle in combat without fear of fatigue in dealing with an opponent to the end is a wonderful attribute. Furthermore, when the basic exercise of circle walking is well practiced, it is possible to attack the lesser position with a straight force or to attack the greater position with a force in accordance with the offensive gesture of the opponent for guiding him to enter an empty position and then finishing him. Therefore, close attention should be paid to the following points in practicing circle walking:

1) There are no limitations in the size of the circle and in the direction of walking, ultimately, this is determined by the practitioner. However, for beginners it is advisable to walk eight steps in a circle and to walk as slowly as possible because slow walking can detail correctly the training of the legs.

2) Maintain a sense of orientation. In combat when changing positions, one must keep oriented. The constant changing of positions through left and right turning and circle walking will confuse the opponent producing panic that can lead to his defeat. With long-term practice, dizziness will not be a factor. One can freely observe the opponent while circling and seeking out the weakest point, take the opportunity to attack, and finish him.

3) Remember the standing song, song of the forty-eight methods. "Walking constantly I rely on the principles of the eight diagrams. Each step (posture) depends on changing footwork. Standing still would invite defeat." The circling in Eight Diagram Palm walks suddenly to the East then suddenly to the West. When changing in circle walking, the palmwork, footwork and bodywork automatically change in accordance. These tactics are intended to puzzle the opponent with movement and walking. By standing still one would be set up for defeat and liable to be tread upon by anyone. This would violate the principle of constant change in the Eight Diagram Palm.

4) In circle walking one should be "twisted together like a rope." This would, in effect, pull all the strength in the body together in order to be able to change the gestures in walking and turning and to change the movement of palms for free and skillful application.

Footwork and circle walking in Eight Diagram Palm requires

Characteristics of Eight Diagram Palm

the ability to walk quickly and slowly, to walk lightly and freely, and also to be able to walk gently with strong force. Proper training of the footwork requires strict adherence to these guidelines. This demanding regimen of leg training enables one to embody gentleness within lightness and to appear gracefully soft externally while concealing firm strength in the interior. The skill derived from this training enables the practitioner's footwork to tread with stability, firmness, and nimbleness while maintaining flexibility and liveliness in the waist, arm and palm striking quickly and with agility. Only in this way is it possible to harmonize the three parts, that is, the upper, middle and lower and realize the goal of "the body following the steps to turn, the palms following the body to change and the steps following the palm to turn." This is the method to manifest the form of "walking like a swimming dragon, changing gestures like an eagle and turning the body like a monkey."

In footwork, either the left or the right foot walking forward once is considered one step. The inside foot must walk straight forward; when the outside foot steps on the ground, it must land flat to the ground angled inward so that both of the feet would be in an inward splay-foot form (toed in), which makes it easy to turn and walk in a circle (see illustration and photo on the next page). When either foot steps forward it is necessary to lift the foot flat and step on the ground flat so that neither the heel shows (i.e., lift the heel and drop the toes to show the sole to the rear) nor the anterior part of the sole shows (i.e., lift the toes and show the sole to the front). If either the heel or sole is visible, it would be impossible to stand stable at that point in time and would provide the opponent an opportunity to attack. When changing strokes and gestures, it is important to turn the body and change the gesture only after the anterior foot steps on the ground firmly. It is forbidden to twist the sole or heel like turning a screw. Turning in this manner would cause you to stand less stable with a tendency to sway, again providing an opportunity for the opponent to attack.

The hooking step or *kou bu* is executed by moving the anterior foot inward; both feet being in an inward splay-foot form or T-shaped stance (see illustration and photo on page 11). However, the steps must be small in order to maintain stability and ease in turning. The swinging out step, or *bai bu,* means to swing the anterior foot outward, i.e., turn the toes outward, both feet being in a complex splay-foot form (toed out - see illustration and photo on page 11). Thus, it is easy to turn the body. If walking counter clockwise, *kou bu* step with the right foot is used to turn the body to the left, while the *bai bu* step with the right foot is used

Liang Zhen Pu Eight Diagram Palm

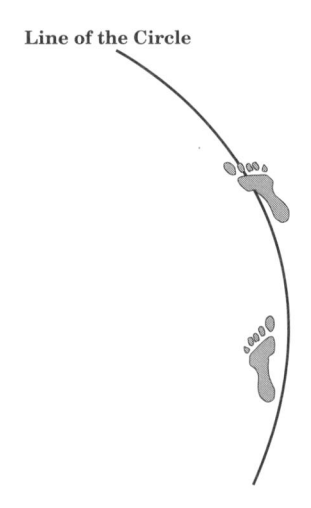

Line of the Circle

Foot Placement in Circle Walking

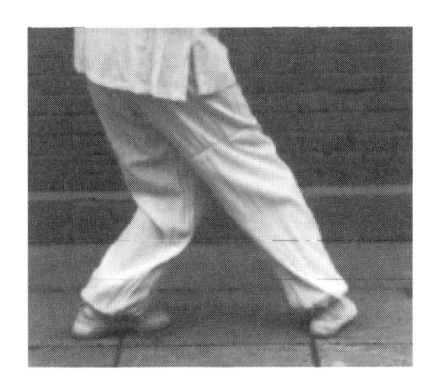

Characteristics of Eight Diagram Palm

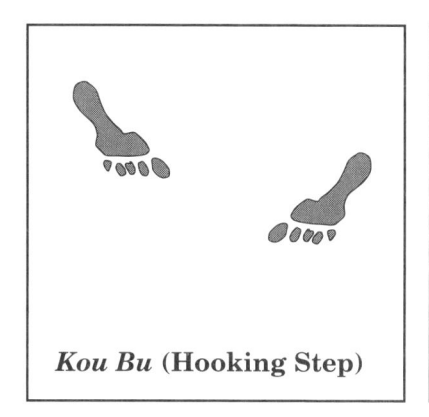

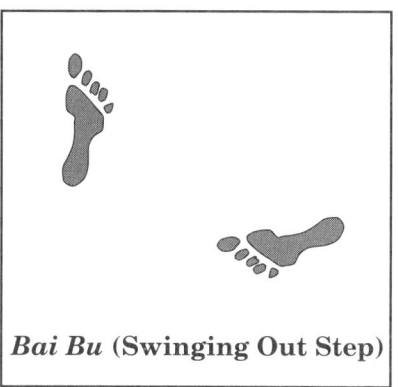

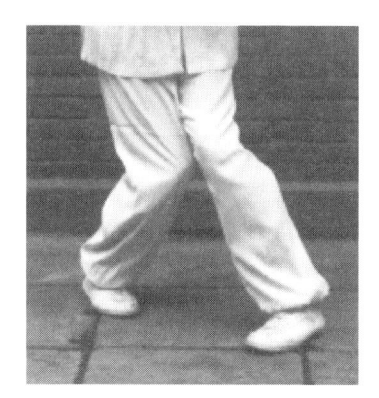

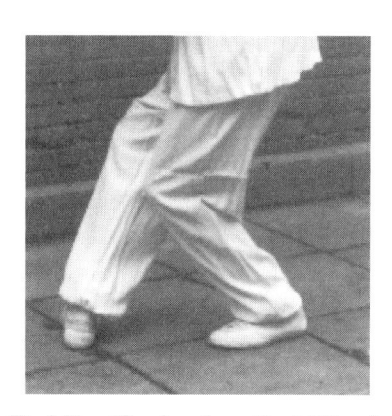

Kou Bu (Hooking Step)   ***Bai Bu*** (Swinging Out Step)

Kou Bu (Hooking Step)   ***Bai Bu*** (Swinging Out Step) to turn the body to the right. The opposite applies on a clockwise circle. Also, no matter which foot moves forward to *kou bu*, both knees must move close together (called rub knees, rub legs or scissor thighs). This protects the groin. When the foot sets on the ground, it should firmly grasp the ground with the toes. This is the so-called "turn foot, close knees and grasp the ground firmly." That is, move the foot inward, close both knees together, set the foot down firmly, and grasp the ground with the toes firmly so that one can stand with stability. When the lower part of the body is stable, one cannot be easily thrown and the opponent is automatically at a disadvantage.

2. Strategy and Tactics of Out Flanking Offenses.

The second characteristic is the use of strategy and tactics based on flanking offensives. When other kinds of boxers engage in combat, most of them would make frontal attacks and move straight forward or backward. This usually results in defeat if the opponent is in a stronger position. Eight Diagram Palm tends to avoid head-on confrontation with an opponent and instead takes the strategy and tactic of out flanking offensives. There are two main reasons for this.

1) When I stand on the lateral side of the opponent, it is easy to observe the opponent's weak points and flaws to attack.

2) This method is a form of guerrilla warfare and as such stresses mobility that is developed and determined by circle walking. But it should be obvious that in practical application the circular walking doesn't proceed in a fixed pattern. It should proceed according to the situation and movements of the opponent, changing and transforming ceaselessly. Whether training or in combat, one moves according to one's opponent. We could decide to attack either the lateral side of the opponent by first moving straight in, or vice versa, in order to induce the opponent to enter an empty position and then defeat him. This is exactly the method of "evading and advancing to win."

The strategy in Eight Diagram Palm may be summarized as attack, defend, advance and retreat. Therefore, it dictates to: "move before the enemy is going to move, be still as the enemy comes to rest,

Characteristics of Eight Diagram Palm

avoid the enemy when he strains, be supple when the enemy is strong and rigid, advance when the enemy retreats, retreat when the enemy advances, move when the enemy moves and also move when the enemy does not move." The military specialists of ancient times had a well-known saying: "long-term defense does not mean victory." We can see that Eight Diagram Palm is one of the boxing methods that applies dialectics for advocating attack. It observes the enemy in movement, changes the postures while moving and achieves victory in movement. All of which expresses the principle of moving when the enemy moves as well as moving when the enemy does not move. This is to say that the attack is the original aim and the defense is only a temporary measure not a permanent solution. Therefore, the Eight Diagram Palm's strategy and tactics are flexible and lively and make use of the palm skills from the eight sets to attack the enemy and defend ourselves, using circle walking as the foundation of attacking and conquering the enemy.

3. Exercise Method Conforms to Natural Principles.

The third characteristic is conforming to natural principles. In order to survive in this world, human beings must live in conformity with natural physiological laws. These laws can be expressed and observed in comprehending the transformational patterns connecting the various sequential stages in the human life-cycle, i.e., birth, childhood, adulthood, decrepitude and death. The Taoist creators of internal school boxing not only understood the laws of natural physiological development but, by mastering those laws, were also able to integrate them in their creation and development of internal boxing skills.

Eight Diagram Palm requires a calm mind, regular breathing and lowering the breath to the Dantian (the area below the umbilicus). Only by conforming to nature, that is, moving naturally, can the respiration be even and regular, the blood circulate smoothly, and the pulse pulsate in rhythm. For promoting physical health, exercise should conform to our physiological nature for regulating metabolism and maintaining a strong and energetic spirit. The practice of Eight Diagram Palm enhances metabolic function and long-term practice will lead to development of the so-called "internal power" (a breaking-out power), which is exactly what practitioners dream about. In combat, this internal power is applied in attacking.

Another aspect of health maintenance is that Eight Diagram Palm, in conforming to the nature of human physiology, strengthens the internal organs enhancing the immune system which provides optimum defense against pathogenic elements. This can have profound ramifications in the pursuit of longevity.

Through the training of the legs with walking and turning as it's basis, Eight Diagram Palm is one of the martial arts that realizes the goal of energy cultivation. So it is very important to develop the energy in the legs and only by doing so can the internal power be cultivated. Therefore, it is necessary to practice the basic exercise of walking the circle diligently, so that one would be able to optimize their development according to the principles of human physiology, promote metabolism and maintain youthful attributes much longer than normally would be expected.

In practice, it is necessary to pay attention to these important details:

1) The lower body is sunken downward while the upper body is held erect.
2) The head is held straight up while the shoulders and elbows are dropped.
3) The back is rounded yet straight and erect while the chest is held in a hollow.
4) The wrists are sunken while the palm remains pressing.
5) The waist is relaxed while the buttocks are tilted up and slightly forward.
6) The knees are flexed with the toes grasping the ground.

Sinking the shoulders and elbows in the upper body will transmit the energy and power to the tips of the fingers. During walking, the feet must move straight forward and step on the ground flat. The body's root is established when the shoulders sink to the waist, the waist sinks to the hip joint, the hip joint sinks to the knees, and the knees sink to the feet. Thus, the energy and power is transmitted to the toes. When it is necessary to change strokes and gestures, there would be no swaying due to this stable stance.

In summary, each part of the body has specific conditions to meet and maintain during the execution of Eight Diagram Palm, but the coordinated synthesis of all these conditions, when performed in synchrony, allows the practitioner to move in a completely natural manner, breathing at ease and moving relaxed. It is in this manner of moving in accordance with the laws of natural physiology that we can cultivate more energy than we expend thereby enhancing one's life force.

The principles of combat in Eight Diagram Palm also originate from natural laws as well. The so-called "hands beat in three and feet kick in seven, all force coming from backward treading of the foot" means that while the hands generate thirty percent of the force applied and the legs generate seventy percent, all of the force ultimately comes through the grounding of the stance and the generation of the force originating from the pressures exerted on the soles of the feet. These principles were developed through prolonged practice and are in complete conformity to the natural laws. The principles are the same as those in Shadow Boxing (*Tai Ji Quan*): "It's root is in the feet, driven up through the thighs, directed in the waist and expressed in the fingers." This is also the so-called "whole power." The power of the thighs is much stronger than that of the hands and the steps will augment the quick actions. Consequently, the Step Stabilizing Song says: "Instability in the steps surely would sway the body, only stepping on solid ground can conquer thousands of gestures." Combined with the nimble turning in the bodywork and the false and true changes in the handwork, one is assured of victory by confounding the enemy's ability to respond. Whether you are practicing the Eight Diagram Palm to improve vitality or to improve boxing skills, the exercises should always conform with natural principles. Practice must proceed slowly and gradually in order to adhere to these natural principles. No haste can be allowed. Beginners especially must practice slowly to secure a good foundation with careful attention to details.

4. Combination of Movement and Stillness and of Firmness and Gentleness.

The fourth characteristic is the combination of movement and stillness and the mutual support of firmness and gentleness. Internal school boxing is characterized by special emphasis on the combination of movement and stillness. In the practice of Eight Diagram Palm the shoulders, waist, hip, knees and feet move, walk and turn constantly. The forward hand extends and the rear hand pushes; the shoulders, elbows and wrists move with the palm. This consolidated moving posture represents stillness in the upper part, while the constant walking in specific contrast represents movement. On the other hand, the swift and complex movement in the changing of gestures and the manipulations of the palms represent movement, while in contrast the

Liang Zhen Pu Eight Diagram Palm

constant and unchanging circle walking represents stillness. This is to say that movement changes and returns to stillness.

In combat, there are no fixed gestures. It is desirable to flank the opponent on one side or the other before moving forward to attack, all according to the gestures of the opponent. This strategy can serve to induce him to enter an empty position, leaving him vulnerable for this attack to better ensure success. For this type of strategy the mind must always be clear and as calm as still water, with free and natural breathing. This is movement on the exterior and stillness in the interior. The calm mind allows for keen vision and quick reaction no matter how fierce the battle, so that one never gets dizzy and the vision never blurs, rendering one as stable as Mt. Taishan.

In terms of physical culture, the combination of movement and stillness maintains a calm mind, deep breathing and a relaxed body, resulting in a harmonious flow of blood and energy to the four limbs, so that the practitioners can train enthusiastically for prolonged periods. By tonifying all the various systems in harmony (i.e., nervous, respiratory, digestive, circulatory, skeletal, and muscular), this training vitalizes the whole body.

The boxing manual of Eight Diagram Palm says: "Movement is the advantage of stillness, and stillness is hidden within movement." In general, the stillness factors (i.e. holdings) develop the physical factors (i.e., strength of postures, etc.) while movement addresses the tactical aspects of combat (i.e., speed, maneuvering, etc.). Therefore, movement and stillness must be combined together.

The strategies and tactics of Eight Diagram Palm were developed upon the theory of changing the palms in accord with the theories of the *Tai Ji* (yin/yang) and the *Ba Gua* (eight transformations). As such, it emphasizes the deficiency and excess of yin and yang, the mutual interpromotion and interaction of the five element theory (*wu xing*), the mutual support of gentleness and firmness, and the unity of the opposites.

In terms of the spiritual energy[1], the exchange of firmness and gentleness is manifested by their storage and release in an unending transformational process. When the power is retained and stored, it would appear gentle and soft (winding up or setting up), while the release of power (discharge) and the use of the force appears strong and firm. The soft or gentle expression is generally applied into the pivotal point in the changing of gestures, while when placing a strike, it is necessary to use firm force, the absence of which would be insufficient to defeat the enemy. This "firm force" is not necessarily a visible force.

If the mutual support of firmness and gentleness is not enforced, the exclusive use of the firm power would cause the rigid strength to spread through the whole body, which would impede the turning of the body and prevent manifesting firmness in the placement of the strike. If, on the other hand, only gentle power is applied, the energy would disperse and not accumulate in a specific area resulting in a lack of firmness in the placement of a strike. So if softness is used when firmness is needed, the energy would not accumulate when necessary and if firmness is applied when gentleness is needed, the energy could not disperse when necessary. These imbalances prevent the magical effect of the mutual support of firmness and gentleness from manifesting.

In contrast, those who are good at the application of firmness and gentleness would store gentleness for releasing firmness and would release firmness in exact placement like the gesture of a dragonfly skimming the surface of the water. This is the correct image of manifesting firm placement. In every change of the stroke and gesture, the gentle power should be applied like a constant turning wheel. This is the correct image of manifesting the gentle power. Only in this way, can the mutual support of firmness and gentleness be applied with magical effect.

The theory of eight diagrams contains within it the dual dynamics of yin/yang theory as does the transformational construct of the five elements matrix which is comparable to eight diagrams in its application of theory to martial arts. All three of these classical Chinese matrices are, in reality, integrated and superimposed in their application within all of the internal arts.

5. The Eight Contraries.

The fifth characteristic is the eight contraries. Eight Diagram Palm is also called Eight Reverse Palm (*Ba Fan Zhang*). Eight Diagram Palm is one of the last classical martial arts developed in history. It's creators were able to extract from other boxing styles those particular skills that clearly lent to the success of that style but, in fact, conformed to a more generic set of principles common to superior athletic performance as well as combative strategies and tactics in general resulting in a special and distinctive expression of training and performing. The eight contraries are an enumeration of the eight major distinctions that are considered to be the signature of the Eight Diagram Palm. They are as follows:

Liang Zhen Pu Eight Diagram Palm

1) Go forward with the anterior step first, retreat with the posterior step first.

2) Everyone advances forward with a straight step, but we advance on an angle with a twisted step, then walk with a cross step and turn around with a reverse step.

3) Everyone likes to show various gestures, but we just wait to move in the stillness.

4) Everyone likes to use their fists and kick, but we use penetrating palms and hidden elbows.

5) Everyone uses the ends of their limbs, but we use the root first when we want to use the ends.

6) Everyone likes to use varied fists, but we use the straight pushing palm.

7) Everyone likes to turn the whole body around to face the rear, but in a single step we can move to deal with the eight directions.

8) Everyone advances straight forward with the erect body, but we strike with our palm and the feet follow.

The above-mentioned eight contraries are refined with long-term practice and experience of the actual combat. Mr. Dong Hai Chuan said: "The skill of circle walking is the foundation of Eight Diagram Palm. Therefore, it is necessary to consolidate its foundation in practice. Everyone likes to go forward and retreat with the straight steps, but we should go out and around and enter with the twisted steps. Everyone hopes to master the many varied hand skills for attack and defense, but we just push the straight palm to evade an attack." All these aspects require complete understanding in the mastery of the boxing skills and arts of attack and defense. Therefore, a detailed discussion of some of these fine point is most helpful.

In combat, it is necessary to observe the six directions visually and listen to the eight aspects. (The six directions being right, left, front, back, above and below. The eight aspects being the four cardinal directions (north, south, east, west) and the four oblique angles (northeast,

Characteristics of Eight Diagram Palm

southeast, northwest, southwest)). Even if facing only one opponent, it is difficult to effectively deal with him if one is too casual; it is still necessary to watch in all directions. Even in dealing with only one opponent, it is impossible to anticipate each and every attack, which weapon and from which direction. If we just deal with him by the straight step, surely we would not be able to respond to each and every move and would be too slow in combat even if we run in our steps.

The footwork in walking the circle is the main key to conquering the opponent. In circle walking the waist is held according to what is comfortable and may be adjusted according to the needs of the situation. The anterior foot in circle walking becomes the posterior foot, the anterior hand becomes the posterior hand, and the posterior foot is then moved as the anterior foot and the posterior hand is extended as the anterior hand. This is the principle of change. All of these postures and gestures, such as left spinning and right turning, right spinning and left turning, the front protected to be the back, the back pushed as the front, the thousands of forms in turning and spinning and different changes in defense and offense, are always consistent in the principle that the body is uniform, with the difference being expressed either to the left or right. On examination, these principles of movement and stillness and determination of direction are essential and indispensable with all of them being based on principles of reason and practicality.

In summary, walking the circle is a specific exercise in Eight Diagram Palm, which has its specific function. For example, to go forward first with the anterior foot and to retreat first with the posterior foot are the methods for the quick attack and retreat. In other boxing skills, the straight step is often used for attack and retreat, but we use the twisted step, the striding step and the backward step. It is required, tactically, to circle around the front of the enemy for attacking the lateral side of the enemy and also to enable us to move and turn nimbly causing the enemy to become disoriented and unable to respond accordingly. In ordinary boxing skills, cuffing and kicking, running and jumping look very impressive, but we always insist on the principle of waiting to move in the stillness, which is also the method "to deal with the thousands of changes by no change."

In ordinary boxing skills, usually the hand is clenched in a fist for attack. In punching with the fist, they tend not to use the whole power of the waist and thighs. They only use the power from a portion of the body, which is described as using the " tip." In contrast, Eight Diagram Palm uses penetrating power of the palm to strike with the wrist, which seems to be comparatively stronger than the ordinary boxing skills.

Liang Zhen Pu Eight Diagram Palm

Also, in comparing the palm and the fist, the palm is longer than the fist.

In application of power, it is necessary to use the force from the foot to the thigh and then to the waist and hand. To strike the opponent with unified strength is more powerful. When one with only ordinary boxing skills challenges more than one opponent at a time, he can deal only with the enemy in front of him. If he wants to deal with the enemy behind him, he has to turn his body around. But, the practitioners of Eight Diagram Palm, because of the nimble and active changes in the footwork, need to take only one step in order to deal with enemies from any direction. This is due to the sophisticated designs and strategies in Eight Diagram Palm maneuvering. Consequently, it is possible to have the step and the palm arriving simultaneously or to have the palm followed by the step. But, the key to conquering the enemy still relies upon the nimble and variable footwork in combination with movement and stillness.

In summary of the above five aspects, Mr. Dong Hai Chuan enumerates three definite ways to fight against the enemy:

1) When anyone attacks, I can neutralize it and then strike back at the same time. This is called the Mutual Advance Method.

2) When anyone attacks, I intercept it and strike back at the same time. This is called the Stop and Intercept Method, i.e. to break the attack and to attack back simultaneously.

3) When anyone attacks, I evade and redirect it with footwork. This is called escaping and "melting away" or "melting like a shadow."

His conclusion: "Of the three ways, the first is better than the second. While the third way is the most complicated and profound and can be used only when the technique has been developed to a level of mastery."

The creator of Eight Diagram Palm understood the effectiveness of striking to the heart when attacking opponents. Therefore, when the enemy attacks, it is important for us to protect our center (heart) as well, by turning the body. Strategically, the goal is to evade the real attack of the opponent while seeking a vulnerable spot to counter attack. For these reasons, Eight Diagram Palm skills have been developed with

Characteristics of Eight Diagram Palm

walking and turning as its basic form. Tactically, there are multiple reasons for this walking and turning. The walking itself protects you and meanwhile allows you to observe the enemy. By walking, you avoid a head-on confrontation with the enemy by flanking the lateral side or the back of the enemy in order to attack him. By walking, we can moderate the attack of the enemy by restricting him to fewer offensive options and wearing him down, while we wait to move from stillness, wait at our ease for an exhausted opponent. Then, discovering the opponent's weak spot we can attack and bring him down. Therefore, walking in Eight Diagram Palm is not just ordinary walking and the entire system itself relies on one basic movement - walking. There is a saying: "Hundreds of exercises are not as good as simply walking, walking is the master of hundreds of exercises."

Liang Zhen Pu Eight Diagram Palm

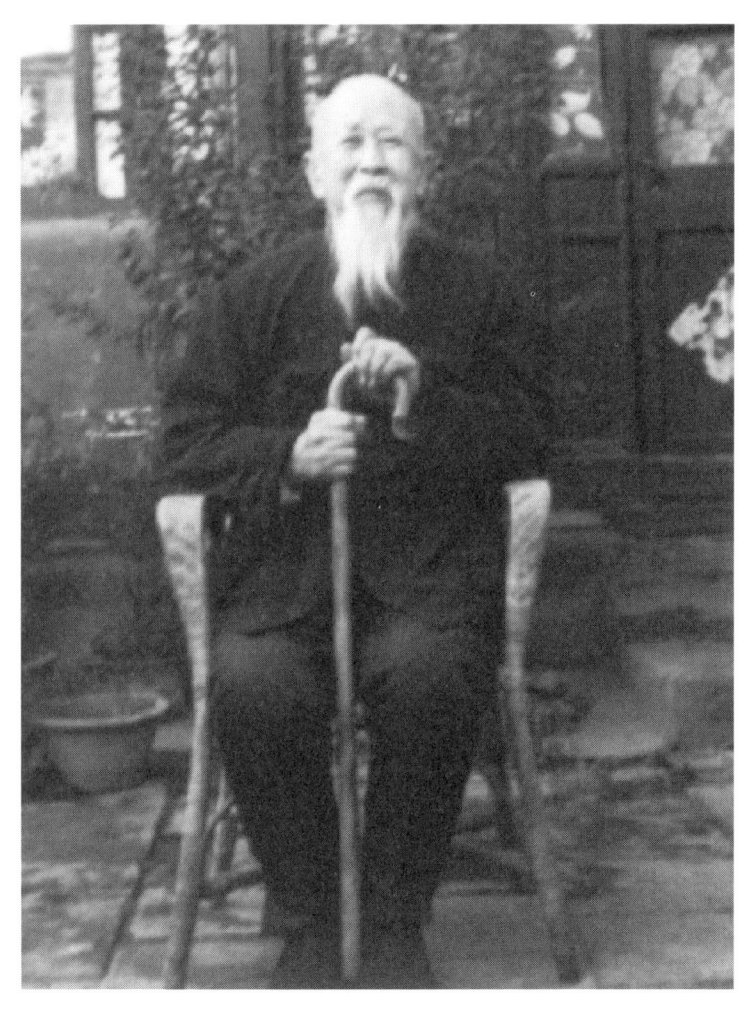

Eight Diagram Palm Master Li Zi Ming, Beijing, 1989

CHAPTER III

SOME MAIN POINTS IN PRACTICE OF EIGHT DIAGRAM PALM

1. Careful Prevention of Three Fatal Errors.

The first main point is to carefully avoid the three harms[1]. A distinguishing feature of internal boxing methods is the emphatic avoidance of training in conflict with certain natural laws of physiological development. It is held in internal boxing that infractions of these laws in long-term practice will result in harmful development and possibly serious consequences. The three harms or harmful habits to avoid are:

1) *Holding the breath or oppressed breathing.* This can cause a stuffy and distending sensation, damaging the lung and it's energy. Therefore, one should stay mindful that the breathing is always free and natural and unrestrained.

2) *Labored use of strength.* This describes holding power or holding a single part of the body rigid in order to exert force. Holding in this way one tends to use only the local power of the hand and the foot, not applying the full synergy of the whole body power, so that it would negatively influence the blood circulation and lead to stagnation of blood in the local areas[2]. This often leads to holding or oppressed breathing as well.

3) *Throwing out the chest and sucking in the abdomen.* This can lead to stasis of the energy in the lung which then fails to descend to the Dantian area. Because the energy is blocked, it cannot flow through the whole body. This results in upward floating of the energy and, consequently, the center of balance of the body would tend to ascend, leading to a lack of root and instability in the stance.

These three bad habits must be carefully eschewed due to their not conforming to the natural laws of physiological development. But, early on in practice there is a strong tendency to hold the breath and hold the power (strain), which is usually due to anxiety related tension. The tendency to throw out the chest and lift the abdomen must be gradually corrected by persistent and exacting practice. In daily life, the practitioner should always maintain an erect posture, pressing up with the crown, dropping the shoulders and elbows, holding the spine erect, hollowing the chest, relaxing the waist and hip whenever walking, standing, sitting or sleeping. At the same time, one should cultivate a habit of reverse breathing[3] to insure the energy always descends to the Dantian area.

Avoiding these bad habits allows a calm mind and even breathing, and keeps the energy in the Dantian area. This creates an empty sensation in the chest and a full sensation in the abdomen for stable and natural walking and turning. This allows for carefree and satisfying training. This manner of training will gradually strengthen the physical constitution and increase the internal power.

2. Combination of Attack Skill and Art.

The second main point is combining the aforementioned principles with the attacking skills in an artful manner. Boxing skills are the basis of the Chinese martial arts. They are the precise method applied to contend with the enemy. At the same time, it is also a method to enhance the physical constitution. Therefore, the training method should integrate the skill of a combative challenger and the refined expression of a dancer. Eight Diagram Palm does precisely this. Correct practice requires light and nimble movements, free and spontaneous turning in mid-action, and a whole body power above and below (unity of motion), in order to effect free application of boxing skills in an actual situation.

At the same time, many movements are based on the specific characteristics of various animals. These movements are relatively complex and the images and characteristics of the animals must be manifested in practice. These movements and their names together produce powerful and picturesque images, such as Lion Rolling Ball, White Snake Protruding Tongue, Hawk Shooting through the Sky, White Ape Offering Fruits, Blue Dragon Turning Body, Lion Shaking Head, Unicorn Spitting Soil, Swallow Skimming Water, Huge Boa Turning Body, Roc Spreading Wings and Black Bear Turns Back

Some Main Points in Practice

Around. These movements should manifest continuously while walking and turning. For example, composite images of "walking like a dragon, while changing postures like an eagle, and moving and twisting like a monkey," or "moving like a dragon, crouching like a tiger, and moving and turning like a lion rolling a ball" allows us to imbue many qualities into two or three movements in a flowing and continuous expression. To be effective in the attack art, it is also required to "move like the wind and stand as if nailed in place." It is not easy to embody the above-mentioned images and can only be achieved through long-term, meticulous training.

When all the skills are masterfully polished, it is possible to attack and retreat freely, to disintegrate the strokes of the enemy, while delivering ones own strokes; enabling one to be firm without being stiff and relaxed without being limp. The resultant stability would produce the stillness of Mt. Taishan while allowing ceaseless movement like the rivers. Twisting and coiling, turning and circling, each movement conceals many strikes. Therefore, one would be able to change at any time according to the actual situation in combat. Attaining this level of performance is an extraordinary experience, calm in the mind and comfortable in the body and smooth in the hundreds of meridians, so that the heart can feel at ease throughout. This results in the enemy becoming puzzled in mind, deranged in spirit and thereby defeated in battle. This is a kind of specific effect produced by the proper blending of the attack skills and the artistic images in Eight Diagram Palm.

Nowadays some people emphasize only enhancing the health and speak nothing of the attack skills in their practice and teaching of the boxing method. I suspect this bias is due to the lack of knowledge of the actual boxing skills and their indispensable importance to the further development of optimum health. These boxing skills are the substance from which Chinese martial arts are created. The martial arts are precisely this, the attacking and defensive skills of mortal combat. Therefore, the arts of attack must be emphasized in the practice of boxing. Otherwise, the essentials of the boxing skills would be omitted and the significance of the Chinese martial arts would be lost. The boxing would become just another kind of dance or exercise.

In order to preserve the original purpose of the Chinese martial arts, it is essential that the practitioners research the arts of attack. In order for the practitioners to ensure correct gesturing, it is essential they perfect the arts of attack. The martial arts research is exactly that, research of the attacking skills. Only when the principles of attack and defense are completely understood is it possible to have correct gesturing through which we achieve maximum benefit to the body's vitality. So, again, the arts of attack must be stressed. Some people may presume that the training of the attack arts makes one more eager to fight. Those who hold this prejudice do not understand a basic precept of internal boxing, i.e., in a quarrel with somebody, we would never move first to strike the first blow; even when attacked by an opponent, we would not counter attack unless absolutely necessary.

Presently, around the world the Chinese martial arts are highly regarded. Associations and organizations of the Eight Diagram Palm have been established for further research in many countries. However, since China was the birthplace, China can never neglect the research of the attack arts and must always preserve this creation of our ancestors and all its subsequent advancements. This body of knowledge should be carried forward and handed down completely and systematically as a national treasure of China.

3. Guidelines for Practice.

The third main point is to obey the guidelines for practice. It is necessary to remember and follow the strict formula which articulates the specific requirements for the various parts of the body in the practice of Eight Diagram Palm. The main requirements are:

The head should be straight and erect, with intention pushing the head up. The neck should be erect with the chin slightly moved inward. This will enhance the neck position. The two eyes look straight forward and the tongue curls to touches the upper palate, with intention pressing the upper palate. The shoulders should sink in relaxation and not be shrugged but be held slightly inward.

The elbows should drop and not raise up. The palm should be straight and erect with five fingers apart and the wrist should drop down. The finger tips should be extended forward slightly. The thumb is slightly curved, the index finger and the middle finger must point upward, the ring finger and the little finger must be together so that the area between the thumb and the index finger can be spread and rounded. This creates a slight hollowing in the center of the palm. Both arms, whether forward or rear, should maintain a slight curve. The arms cannot be extended completely straight without losing the curved quality in the elbow position. Neither should the arms flex too much lest

Some Main Points in Practice

they form too much of a triangle. This is known as "the dead curve." The two arms should also have the intention of "embracing."

The chest should be relaxed inward and the back slightly rounded. This will allow the smooth passage of energy and facilitate the energy's descent to the lower abdomen (Dantian). Do not throw out the chest or hold in the abdomen. The waist must be relaxed and sunken while the hips should be relaxed and lifted. Only in this way can one walk and turn lightly and nimbly and still turn the upper body freely. Otherwise, it would be awkward and difficult to turn the body, preventing the waist from being the axis. When the buttocks are pulled in and the pelvis is lifted, it forms a vertical line from Pt. Baihui (GV20) on the vertex, to Pt. Huiyin (CV1) at the tip of the coccyx, stabilizing the whole body forward and backward.

The thighs should squat down, but a triangle should not be formed by the thighs, calves and knees, there must be curve to the structure, or else it will be a "dead bow" or stiff. The knees should be close for shifting the gravity[4] below the shoulders to the waist, the waist to the hip, and the hip to the thighs and then further to the knees and feet. This is the so-called "Four Drops." Sinking the gravity of the body to the thighs and legs, allows the upper body to be nimble and reduces the likelihood of being thrown or falling down. When the gravity is in the lower part, because the two knees are closed, the knees should rub each other when walking, which is described as "rubbing knees and ankles." With the knees close together, the legs in walking and turning resemble a scissor action and, therefore, are also called the "scissor thighs." The closed knees also serve to protect the crotch.

During practice, both feet should lift and step down flatly without exposing the heel or the sole. In stepping forward, the dorsal surface of the foot should be extended out flat so that the toes do not rise higher than the heel. When the posterior foot is lifted, first lift the great toe and then lift the posterior foot. In this way, the two feet can walk without showing the heel or the sole. It is also necessary to grasp the ground with the five toes when either foot steps on the ground. This is described as "stepping on the ground and planting the root." In this way the body can be balanced and stable when walking and turning. This manner of walking is as though one were walking in mud. This is the so-called "mud stepping step." Because the five toes grasp the ground, the center of the foot automatically is drawn inward. This is called "hollow of foot"; like the "hollow of heart" and the "hollow of chest." Together they are called "the three hollows."

Practice of Eight Diagram Palm must conform to the above-mentioned formula. This formula and all its regulations are in accord with the principles of physiological performance and necessary for cultivating the internal energy. As one practices patiently and correctly he would gradually adjust to all of these requirements as time goes by. This approach is the path to natural ability. While perfecting the maneuvers of Eight Diagram Palm, the whole body will automatically synchronize to yield the "internal power" that the masters of the Chinese martial arts pursue. In this way, one can develop and maintain physical vitality while improving self-defense skills.

It is important to persistently concentrate on the Dantian area during practice. In moving the palms, it is advisable to apply intention rather than physical force (i.e. tension) on the palms. The proverb says: "The heart is the marshal, the eyes are the scout, the feet are the warhorse and the hands are the weapons." The eyes have the observation function, while the hands have the turning and pulling abilities, the feet have the ability to quicken the speed, and the mind, ultimately, has the overall governing control. Therefore, in practice, it is necessary to have the hand following the mind and step following the hand, push the palm like an ox tongue and change the palm like a moving shuttle. In releasing power, it is advisable to have the mind following the eyes, the energy following the mind and the physical force following the energy. The power should be released from the feet to the thighs, to the waist and, finally, to the hand. In this manner, the power can be released quickly and with a whole body synergism. When the whole body power is applied, there must not be any unnecessary rigidity so that the hand can deliver the strength of the body accurately, as well as powerfully.

To enhance the physical vitality, as well as improve self-defense skills, requires proper understanding of the relationships of the four ends and the nine sections. In practice, it is necessary to consciously guide the energy and blood to reach the four ends. Expanding on this, it is said: "The four ends should be equal in length"[5], and the formula is that the tongue presses as if it supports the teeth, the teeth clench as if to brace the tendons, the nails as if penetrating the bones and the hair as if standing on end seems to push away the hat. If force is used in the four ends rather than through them, it would change their length. This would reveal itself in unbalanced dynamics and looks terrible. The four

Some Main Points in Practice

ends are the exit points of the internal power originating in the root. Regarding the nine sections, the body is divided into three sections and each section is further divided into three more sections, totalling nine sections in all. "In regards to the body as a whole, the head is the tip section, the body trunk is the middle section and below the waist is the root section. Regarding just the arm, the hand is the tip, the arm is the middle section and the shoulder is the root. Regarding the lower limb, the foot is the tip, the thigh is the middle section and the hip is the root." The release of power in internal boxing originates in the root, goes through the middle section to reach and exit through the tip. Therefore, the saying that "when the tip is to be used, first apply the root" must be remembered in regards to the four ends and nine sections.

Endnotes

[1]Also called the three poisons. The bracketing of the three harms emphasizes the fine distinction between the external school of thought and the internal school of thought. It recognizes the problematic nature of physically performing according to internal monitors and other mechanisms.

[2]This can be witnessed in the so-called pumping up of energy exercises in external systems of athletic endeavor resulting in sore, aching muscles for several days following an excessive work out as well as extremely tight muscles and reduced flexibility.

[3]Reverse breathing is a technique in which one draws the abdomen inward while inhaling and drawing the breath down to the abdomen being careful not to unduly expand the upper thoracic area. On exhalation the abdomen relaxes and expands with air. This serves to direct the *Qi* down to Dantian.

[4]The gravity he is referring to is the root in the sense of projecting your center of balance to a lower relative position of the body for ballast and power.

[5]The phrase "equal in length" connotes the necessity of simultaneous connection to the four ends in such a manner that when the whole body power is generated and applied, it manifests equally in all of the extremities. This results in an internally balanced bracing of the body's physical structure in the expression of that power. In this action all the body parts, in effect, begin and end their movement at the same time so that visually all parts of the body would stop at the same instant.

Liang Zhen Pu Eight Diagram Palm

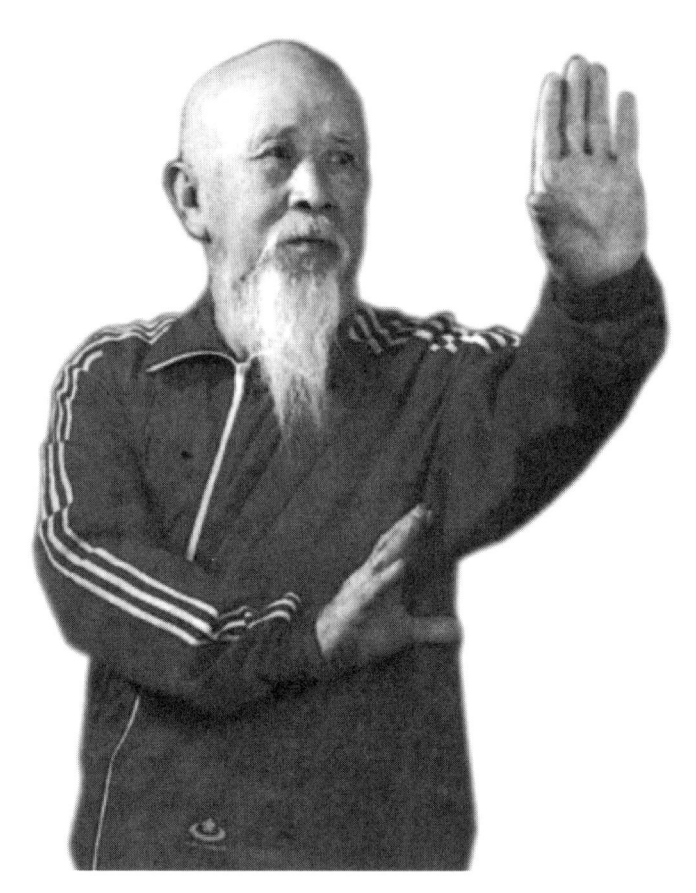

"*It is hard to advance on the enemy in a true fight,
But all is possible with vigorous power in
eyes that are bright.*"

CHAPTER IV

COMPILATION OF THEORY ON EIGHT DIAGRAM PALM

For easy memorization and convenient application, all types of academic theories in China's ancient times were compiled into rhymed songs or formulae, such as the multiplication table in arithmetic and rhymed songs of the herbal formulae in traditional Chinese medicine. All internal and external Chinese martial arts have their own respective sets of formulae for guidance in practice. In earlier times, due to the different schools of thought and prejudice among the different kinds of martial arts, these formulae were not so easily accessible to everyone. In order to ensure the flourishing development of Eight Diagram Palm and benefit the health of all people, I have compiled these rhymed[1] formulae handed down by our senior masters. They are as follows:

1. Sixteen Word Formula of Eight Diagram Palm

The first formulation: Push, hold up, bring, guide, remove, close off, chop, advance, penetrate, dodge, cut off, block, touch, connect, stick and follow.

The second formulation: Penetrate, remove, cut off, block, twist, overturn, walk, rotate, push, hold up, bring, guide, entwine, hook, close off and drill.

These sixteen words simply list sixteen different ways, or specific techniques, to apply power.

Liang Zhen Pu Eight Diagram Palm

2. Formulae of Hand, Eye, Body, Method and Step

Every style of boxing emphasizes it's own specifics in application of hand, eye, body, method and footwork. Eight Diagram Palm has its own particular emphasis as well. Masters know these formulae well but students must write them and eventually commit them to memory. Now, I write them down here as reference for the students.

1) Formula of Starting Gesture

*The body is erect in the standing posture with the palm
used like a fist,
Yin and Yang are in their proper place.
Observe gesture clearly, knowing when to dodge,
Protect the body's flanks by observing the limits.
Advance, press, and uplift with stealing step footwork[2],
 Perfectly insert, strike, split and penetrate.
To avoid confusion of the mind and hands in the actual situation,
And meticulously study these songs with patience.*

2) Formula of Hand

*Use groin strike and uplifting palm like wind and smoke,
Split, penetrate, grasp and seize are all valuable skills.
Execute in lateral direction.
The feet step firm in advance and retreat,
Hooking, removing, binding, pulling, slicing and splitting one
after the other.
Meticulously develop internally and externally the three parts of
the body,
Strike all directions, front, back, high and low.
Training three years this way without resting even one day,
 One easily can overturn a mountain just by extending a hand.*

3) Formula of Eye

The eyes open wide like bright stars,
For the head to observe the gestures more clearly.
Guard ahead and mind behind glancing quick as lightning,
The body moves and turns like a wheel.
Continually watch the enemy's body, hand and foot,
Seek the chance and do not hesitate in attacking.
It is hard to advance on the enemy in a true fight,
But all is possible with vigorous power in eyes that are bright.

4) Formula of Body

The head and face are upright with hands extended apart,
The body is erect and the thighs protect the crotch.
The feet stand apart in a splay-foot position,
Like riding a horse and stretching a bow.
When the feet and thighs do not float, the body is stable,
The feet step down flat for maneuvers active and nimble.
The heel advances and retreats together with the foot,
And the waist and buttocks move with the shoulders.
Relax the body immediately after turning the body and pull the abdomen in,
So that dodging and leaping in evasion will come easy,
 Practice as if fighting with many enemies,
Ceaselessly attacking to the side and smashing straight ahead.

5) Formula of Method

The profundities hide deeply and mysteriously,
Boxing palm can only be taught by a master and
learned through attentive study.
Hundreds of palm methods, it is impossible to learn all,
Hundreds of tricks difficult to explain.
Where water flows, a channel would appear after three years,
Steel must be smelted before it can cut solidity.
In general, practice makes perfect,
Everything is mutually influenced and connected.

6) Formula of Foot

Both knees flexed with natural force,
Advance in flexibility and retreat in straitness for practicing as solidly as possible.
In zig-zagged walking, dodge following smooth movement and jump to move steps,
In complicated zig-zagged walking, attack obliquely then return to the circle.
The shoulders stay down and level even when spinning and overturning,
With strong knees, straight heels and curved legs.

3. Circle Walking Song of Eight Diagram Palm

Circle walking relies upon Yin and Yang,
Five elements and six harmonies.
Seven stars and eight steps form nine palaces,
One distinguishes firmness and gentleness internally and externally in the three levels of the body.
All unites into one energy on a supporting foundation,
Four aspects and four angles stabilize eight directions.
The body follows the kou bu steps,
Release force in the four tips and magnify energy by turning and walking.
The forward palm extends like an ox tongue in its false and true gestures,
The rear hand below the elbow keeps.
Advance in orderly ways and retreat with methods,
Change and turn the palm in Yin and Yang.
Oblique seems the front in erect and straight, transverse and flexion,
Turning and rotation in circling is controlled by the waist and hips.
Internally, five elements are expressed in the tips,
Externally the five elements are distinguished through observation.
Internally the Qi travels to all three sections,
Externally the hand methods are distinguished in Yin and Yang.
Walking the circle is separated into eight directions,
In body movement pay attention to intent and Qi.
Be supple in turning and changing, do not stop to hold postures,
Yield infinite power high, low, far and near.
The waist movement coordinates the four tips,
The eyes watch eight directions.

Liang Zhen Pu Eight Diagram Palm

The handwork harmonizes with changing situations,
Applications change appropriately to protect left and right.
The shoulderwork should be harmonized in the change of Yin and Yang,
The bodywork should harmonize so rotation is strong.
The hipwork should be harmonized to get close to the opponent,
The kneework should harmonize close to the side of his body.
The footwork should harmonize in rapid retreat and advance,
The strength of the waist and hips permeate dodging, extending, leaping, and shifting.
In the head strike the intent leads the movement and the force comes from the waist and hips,
When rising and falling, maintain central equilibrium.
The feet bring you into the opponent's center gate so that you stand in a superior position,
The palm thrusts straight out in piercing palm, striking quickly high and low.
When the opponent's palm strikes, the lead hand protects the head,
While the elbow strikes with the intention of piercing the chest.
The back stays stretched, the chest remains relaxed and the grain duct is pulled up,
The shoulder and hip both strike with Yin and Yang confluence.
Containing the Qi relies on correct bodywork,
Both hands remain in front of the chest.
Pushing, pressing up, leading, and guiding; all follow the body's force,
Move away, close off, split and advance quickly high and low.
The eight postures and eight fundamental palms originate from continuous turning,
Use palm techniques as a basis for understanding spear and sword.
If one studies the traditional writings one can understand the

Compilation of Theory

theory of Eight Diagram Palm,
If one applies the theory martially, one can understand the principle of change and be victorious.
Boxing skills of senior masters are passed down today,
But very seldom can common people grasp the truth.
Don't blame the conservative ideas of ancestors,
Just regret that we have not practiced our martial arts enough.
To fathom the logic and comprehend the theories,
One realizes that if a tree has luxuriant leaves and branches its roots must go deep.
Eight Diagram Palm skills start with circle walking,
It is only by thoroughly investigating this method can one realize its true utility.
Erect the head, drop the shoulders and flow energy downward,
Direct Qi to the Dantian area for even out-flow and in-flow.
The arm is divided into three sections for practical application,
The bodywork must be equally expressed in the four tips.
The circle around which one walks is separated into eight directions, each represented by a character,
The hand and body move together and all is filled with vitality.
Contract and lift the anus to hold the primordial Qi,
The arms extend like an ape's, the back is broad like a bear's, the body moves with the power of a tiger and supple grace of a dragon.
When facing an opponent it is advisable to seek the wrist,
Move the hands and find advantage in the footwork.
Move up, down, back, forth, right, and left moving to the inside and the outside striking with the shoulders, elbows, knees, and hips.
Extend the thigh without it being seen,
In Eight Diagram Palm, from beginning to end, the thigh is the root.
In Thirty-six movements, front, back, right and left,

The foot moves diagonally and raises smoothly with certainty.
Advance and retreat, hook and lift with obvious and hidden leg work,
Continuously interchanging Yin and Yang while turning the body.
Stomping, thrusting to the side, kicking straight out with the heel, whirling about, bending, piercing, tripping,
All of these one may use as one pleases when they are trained to perfection.
Even if one is highly skilled in martial arts, one must still teach methodically to prevent the student from wasting his time and exerting himself for not,
While skills are obtained in learning martial arts,
They are developed in proper order so one skill does not impede the development of another,
Everyone respects outstanding skill,
When the learning process is at a high level,
One will surpass all others.

4. Song of Eight Diagram Palm Walking About the Circle

Eight diagram continuous palms are divided by five elements,
Showing infinite changes in the creative and destructive cycles.
Six harmonies functioning as one is the real root,
With distinctive separation of Yin and Yang.
Qian evolves from Xun and goes into Li and Kun,
Gen moves to Kun and comes from the same origin as Zhen and Dui.
Move through the eight gates, first straight then oblique, squarely ahead, then reversing,
Spring forward obliquely and ram straight ahead maneuvering back and forth and side to side as one pleases.

Compilation of Theory

The footwork for the palm method is derived from the nine palaces,
Yielding precise changes in left and right rotation of the body.
Striking with or against the opponent's movement, hands moving with the body,
Step in advance and retreat, coordinating the four tips.
The foot kicks undetected,
While the palm strikes without warning.
In turning and rotating the body the postures are never set,
Executing footwork to four corners and four sides one is impenetrable.
One can extend to strike far away or hit at close range,
The footwork of five elements brings about this miraculous effect.
Of the thirty-six stratagems, evasion is the best plan,
Strike no pose, hold no posture, leave no opening.
Strikes should move out from the body,
It is skillful for the hand and foot to arrive together.
The body is like a strong bow and the hand is like an arrow,
The power is derived from the thrust of the rear leg.
Walking without form and stepping without a shadow,
Move like a whirlwind.
Never raise the hand or place the foot without purpose,
Dodge side to side to defend left and right,
Technique will flow of its own accord and move high and low as the situation demands.
Coming and going follow the opponent's body to change,
With the foot beating seven and hand three.
Heavy blows and relentless advance would bring about quick victory,
However, one who is supple can deflect and gain the upper hand.
Use of all three sections of the arm in striking indicates skill,
One sees neither shadow or shape in the ceaseless onslaught.
The body revolves continuously moving left and right, to the side

and straight in with ease.
Evade like a wild cat and advance like a tiger,
Kicking and stomping without error.
Advance undetected,
Strike without palm or fist being seen.
Move the hands and feet automatically without conscious action,
As if in a dream.
There are no feints in combat, it is a game of inches,
He who strikes first wins.
Know the steps for coming in and going out when extending the palm,
Move away like water and advance like wind.
Don't waste steps in leaping and jumping about,
Use distinct handwork for effective dodging, extending and evading.
If stepping hastily, turn using scissor step,
Be distinctive in the seven step striking method.
Leaning to the side or wobbling results from stepping incorrectly,
It is also an error to lean the body forward and backward.
The foot and fist should arrive in unison without telegraphing,
If you cannot do this, your skills are not developed.
The sleeping Dragon is awakened by thunder,
Strong winds bend the limbs of even great trees.
Take precautions internally by keeping stable externally,
Discern the false and true of the situation.
One hand can be used as eight hands,
To move continuously and economically takes real skill.
Thousands of strokes are not equal to one excellent stroke,
Ten thousands strokes are no better if not effective.
Two arms can do the job of many hands,
Real skills are shown by proficient use of the elbows.
To comprehend this peerless system,
One succeeds where ever he goes.

Compilation of Theory

5. Song of Eight Diagram Palm Applications

The palm is divided into eight gestures with rotation as its root,
It is necessary to contract the body in left and right rotation.
Seek out the wrists in a fight between two people,
Victory in fighting depends on use of footwork.
It is necessary to learn the truth of the mysterious eight diagrams,
Walking, piercing, twisting and overturning make it difficult for the enemy to penetrate.
No matter how great his force, as he attacks I evade by turning and revolving to get close to his side.
Eight forms in eight diagrams are produced by Yin and Yang,
With the truth hidden in sixty-four palms.
When tendons and bones are developed intensely,
Qi can run through the body, flowing transversely and vertically.
Congenital Qi needs to be cultivated,
For the combination of firmness and gentleness to be carefully researched.
Knowing palm methods of the eight diagrams by heart,
One need not fear a brutal enemy.
Externally, pay attention to hand, eye, body, method and foot,
Internally, cultivate spirit, mind and will.
Cultivate internal energy with ascending, descending, opening and closing movements,
If there is treasure in the Dantian area, the mystery can be infinite.
To have hun and haa in conjunction with sucking and spitting,
Can shock the opponent like a thunderbolt.
Qian, Kun, Gen and Xun are divided into four corners,
Kan, Li, Zhen and Dui complete the eight diagrams.
It is necessary to understand the mystery of the three steps in the practice of skills,
The Qi of the upper and lower cannot separate from the center.

Liang Zhen Pu Eight Diagram Palm

*Eight Diagram Palm holds the training of the three parts paramount,
Three parts and three sections are further divided into three.
The skills of three parts rely upon the legs,
With mud stepping footwork and concentration on the Dantian.
The three Dantian's are mutually supported by water and fire,
Forceful power of the palm flows from Yangquan (K1).
Painstakingly practice the art to uncover the mystery,
Understanding of its doctrines can foster longevity.
Seek firmness in gentleness,
The skill lies in small movements, continuity, pliability and softness.
The power of nine sections can be realized,
By understanding of the principles.
Palm, fist, elbow and wrists,
Shoulder, waist, hip, knee and foot.
Hand, eye, body, method and step,
Are all are components of martial arts movement.
The whole body exerts a unified force,
Which can be obtained gradually from the interior.
Moving left and right the variations are endless,
Move the elbows quicker than a monkey or cat.
Turn with stable steps,
Stand firmly like Mt. Taishan.
Flies and insects cannot light upon you undetected,
While your touch is as light as a goose feather.
If Eight Diagram Palm is studied,
Your skills surpass others.*

6. Song of Eight Diagram Palm

In Eight Diagram Palm, mobility is primary.
Store then release, evade then return,
False and true change inside the steps.
Move like the wind, stand as if nailed in place,
Bai, kou, penetrating, and overturning footwork must be refined.
With the waist as an axis, and the Qi as a flag,
The eyes watch the way, hand and foot first.
Move like a dragon, crouch like a tiger,
Flow like a river and be still like a mountain.
Hands of Yin and Yang, turning upward and downward,
Sink the shoulder and drop the elbow with the energy concentrated in the Dantian.
Having the six harmonies, avoiding dispersion and disturbance,
Energy flows in the whole body naturally.
Kou and bai steps should be precise,
Rotation, change, advance and retreat rely upon the waist.
Hands strike three, feet kick seven,
Extend hand and foot simultaneously, neither arriving late.
Hip strikes walking, shoulder strikes crashing,
The whole body should press in close and the knees can strike without being seen.
Do not block punches and kicks,
The first priority is to close with the opponent.
These several words of mysterious ways are the key to the boxing skills,
It would be useless without using the pure skill.

7. Method of Eight Boxings in Eight Diagram Palm

1) Head

The method of head punch enters the center,
Lean the mountain and detect the acupoints beside two hypochondriums (floating ribs).
Above the breast and below breast,
The head is the king of the palm.

2) Shoulder

One shoulder hits Yang and the other turns Yin,
The lead arm guides the hand to clear the way.
When changing from hand to shoulder, the shoulder must strike accurately,
Life surely dies when the shoulder beats an approaching head.

3) Hand

Extend the hand to grab, strike, seize and hold,
It is real skill when hand and foot arrive together.
The fist is like a cannon while the body bends like a dragon,
The hand extends forward to split the mountain.

4) Elbow

The elbow strikes the three sections without being seen,
It is necessary to be accurate in striking straightly, transversely and obliquely.
In the method of "tiger embracing its head" the intention is on the elbows,
Penetrate the forest to pierce through the heart.

Compilation of Theory

5) Hip

The hip strikes the mid-section with the shoulder following,
The combination of Yin and Yang force can destroy a mountain.
While one hip withdraws, the other hip moves forward,
The body turns like an eagle to change gesture.

6) Knee

It is difficult to anticipate where the knee may strike,
The knee strike can be a life threatening blow.
When kneeing the hip obliquely use force from the ribs,
Like a fierce tiger jumping out of its cage.

7) Foot

Strike with the swiftness of the wind,
The thrust of the back leg serves notice.
Trample the enemy with the foot stepping down,
It would be completely useless if there are no real skills.

8) Leg

Originally there were seventy-two changes in the legwork,
To trap the enemy with kou bu and bai bu steps.
Sweeping downward and punching upward have their respective implication,
Handwork must precede each and every venture.

Endnotes

[1] In the Chinese spoken language most of these songs would have specific rhythm and rhyme which does not carry over easily into English.
[2] Stealing step footwork refers to the use of half steps.

Liang Zhen Pu Eight Diagram Palm

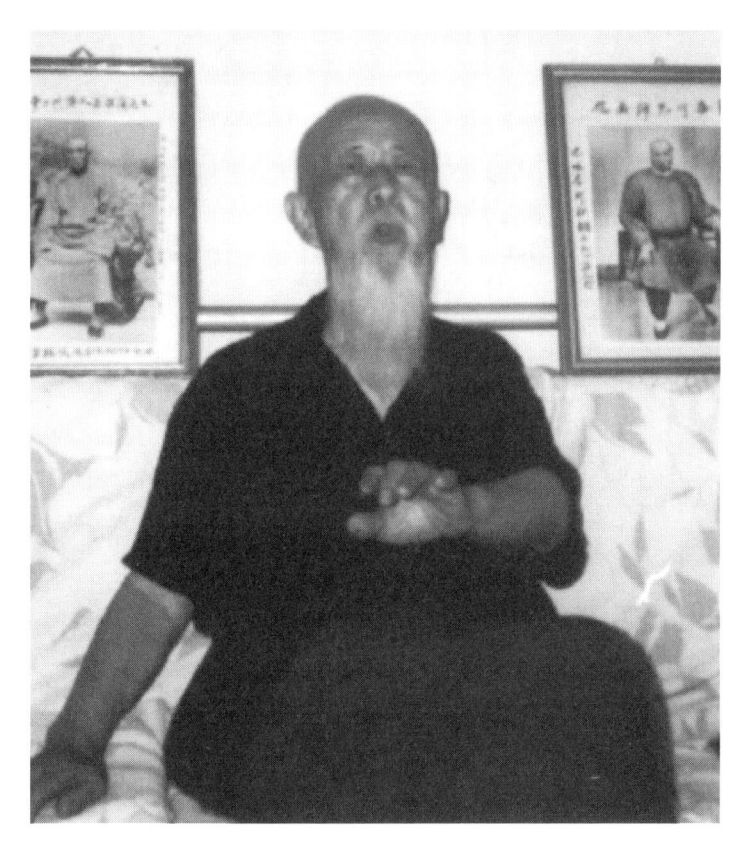

**Li Zi Ming flanked by pictures of his teacher
Liang Zhen Pu and his teacher's teacher,
Dong Hai Chuan**

CHAPTER V

FORMULAE HANDED DOWN FROM MR. DONG HAI CHUAN

The thirty-six formulae for the circle walk practice and forty-eight methods of handwork in Eight Diagram Palm are the unique classic works handed down in the oral instruction by Mr. Dong Hai Chuan. Each sentence of these formulae contains profound significance and puts forth the definite rules for practicing Eight Diagram Palm. These rules pertain to the training of bodywork, rotation of footwork, application of handwork, as well as how to cultivate power, how to move energy and breathe and about what one should be mindful of in fighting against the enemy. These rules cannot be neglected either in cultivation of the physical vitality or in the training for self-defense. Therefore, the practitioners must read these formulae diligently and memorize them, so that they are able to intuit the real mysterious effect of Eight Diagram Palm instinctively. The school of Eight Diagram Palm regarded these formulae as sacred and did not hand them down to people easily. Because the original text of these formulae were composed of special terms and slangs, contemporary scholars would find it very difficult to understand and apply them. Therefore, in accordance with the experience of sixty years of practice in this martial art and with the understanding from instruction of Mr. Liang Zhen Pu, I try to translate them in the following pages. The errors cannot be avoided, I welcome our readers to give suggestions for mutual improvement.

Liang Zhen Pu Eight Diagram Palm

THIRTY-SIX SONGS AND ANNOTATIONS

SONG 1

Hollow the chest, suspend the crown and sink the waist,
Swing the step, join the knees, and grasp the ground firmly.
Sink the shoulders and drop the elbow to extend the forward palm,
The eyes watch between the thumb and the index finger.

Annotation: "Hollow the chest" means to hold the chest in. "Suspend the crown" means to erect the neck and lift the head upward, also called "head lifting suspension." "Sink the waist" means to sink the waist downward in relaxation. "Swing the step" means to move the thighs inward, i.e. in circle walking, move the tip of the lateral foot toward the circle (see illustration on page 10). "Join the knees" means to keep the knees close but without touching each other. "Grasp the ground firmly" means that the toes of the two feet must grasp the ground in walking while stepping on the ground, the so-called "five toes grasping the ground." In this way, the stance is very stable. "Sink the shoulders" means that the two shoulders must drop downward in relaxation. "Drop the elbow" implies to drop the tip of the elbow downward. "Watch between the thumb and the index finger" means that when the eyes watch straight forward, they must focus through the space between the thumb and the index finger.

The first formula is the outline for the practice of Eight Diagram Palm and the basic demands for circle walking in the "millstone pushing" gesture (see photograph on the next page). In the beginning, the practitioners are required to have lifting power in the head, but without tension in the neck, to hollow the chest to round the back, to relax the waist and hip, and to descend the gravity of the body to the two legs for obtaining stability in the lower part of the body. It is also necessary to concentrate on these points fully in training and to train until these conditions are naturally expressed.

"Suspend the crown," also called "pushing up power" or "suspending the vertex", is a method to hold the head straightly erect. When the head is in the erect position, it raises the spirit, radiates a

Formulae

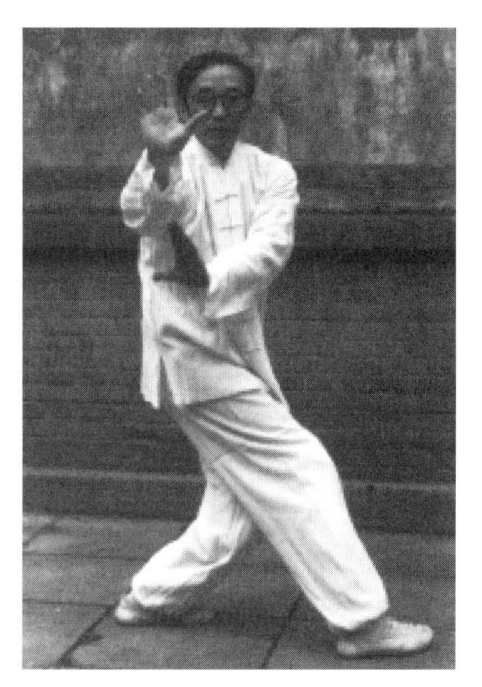

The "millstone pushing" posture

glowing expression of health and vigor, and reflects a shining light in the eyes. Because of the straight erect head, it is easier to hold the body erect. Therefore, the specialists of internal boxing strongly emphasize the straight head and erect body. Only by maintaining this gesture can the movement and turning be lively and nimble.

"Hollow chest and round the back", also called "hold the chest in and pull up the back," is a gesture required by internal boxing. Because the skills of internal boxing are combined with the breathing techniques of the Taoist school, the hollow chest and rounded back are mandatory. If the chest is not hollow and the back is not round, energy cannot return to the Dantian area. Surely, the energy would accumulate in the chest, resulting in full sensation in the chest and shortness of breath. This doesn't conform to the natural laws of physiology, and the resulting shortness of breath would lead to tiring easily. If the energy can be drawn to the Dantian area, the breathing will be deeper and last longer. Therefore, the energy entering the Dantian area is a key to victory in combat, as well as the method for health and longevity.

Liang Zhen Pu Eight Diagram Palm

There is an idiom in Eight Diagram Palm: "Strictly defend four drops." The four drops refer to that the shoulders drop to the waist, the waist drops to the hip, the hip drops to the knees and the knees drop to the feet. That is, sink the shoulders, sink the waist, join the knees, and grasp the ground firmly. When the requirements of the four drops are achieved, one is able to have long, deep breaths that descend to the Dantian area, as well as descend the gravity of the body for secure stability and nimble turning and generate "the internal power." Because the root is planted in the lower part, when striking the enemy the whole body power can be discharged out from the hand after moving up from the center of the foot and through the waist. This is the precise effect of the four drops.

Secondly, the drop of the elbow is a necessary measure for the smooth transmission of power. If the elbow does not drop, the power would stop when it reaches the elbow, and the power could not reach the fingers. Therefore, the elbow must drop downward. At the same time, the drop of the elbow provides protection for the chest and hypochondrium (rib area), and is described as "elbow hiding the heart" in Eight Diagram Palm. Similarly, the rubbing of the knees provide protection to the groin. Therefore, the four drops are a necessary measure to consolidate the lower part. While moving, the waist and hips are supposed to control everything, so that all the actions can be natural and nimble. Hence, the interior and the exterior can match up and the whole body can naturally pull the energy together.

The primary characteristic of Eight Diagram Palm is circle walking. Besides the previously mentioned requirements for gestures, it is also mandatory to have flat rising and flat falling of both feet in circle walking. The so-called "flat rise" means that when the posterior foot is lifted, it is not supposed to show the sole backward. The method is that if the posterior right foot is going to be moved, first move the gravity of the body to the left foot, then lightly hold up the right hip and finally lift starting in the great toe of the right foot. In this way, the right foot can be lifted flat. The so-called flat fall implies that the sole cannot be shown forward when the anterior foot steps on the ground and that the foot must be extended completely before stepping on the ground. After stepping on the ground, the five toes must grasp the ground immediately. It is like walking through wet mud and so it is called "mud step."

If the feet don't rise and flat fall flat, the heel and the sole will be exposed, which violates the principles of Eight Diagram Palm. Because Eight Diagram Palm requirements especially strict upon the thighwork and footwork, it is necessary to have flat rise and flat fall in both feet in

Formulae

order to have stable and quick footwork. When the body squats downward and the knees get closed, the two legs resemble a scissors action in walking and sometimes is called "the scissor thighs." Either with the left rotation or right rotation in walking, the internal foot (closer to the center of the circle) should walk straight forward, and the foot closer to the lateral border of the circle walks with the tip of the foot angled slightly in toward the center of the circle. In this way, the feet become a reverse splay-foot and automatically walk in a circle.

  The waist and hips must rotate toward the center of the circle as much as possible. The waist and hip should also sit down as much as possible. The head is pulled up with the power in the posterior leg. The eyes watch outward over the part between the thumb and index finger of the anterior hand. The shoulder of the anterior hand should be in alignment over the heel of the posterior foot, the posterior hand is slightly curved and held transversely in the front of the chest, with the fingers pointing to the elbow of the anterior hand, while the tip of the finger in the anterior hand should be as high as the eyebrow, and the part between the thumb and index finger should be opened round. Early in training, the steps should be small and the hooking (*kou bu*) and swinging (*bai bu*) movements should be distinctive. During walking, the sole and heel cannot contact with rigid or shocking force. That is to say, the ball or the heel cannot be used as the axis for turning. The *kou bu* and *bai bu* actions can only be done after the whole foot leaves the ground[1]. This is the principle of "step following with the power in the waist, the waist following the step to turn" in Eight Diagram Palm.

    And, finally, attention should always be paid to the mental concentration in adhering to the above-mentioned regulations, so that the eyes, hands, body, feet and methods are applied in close coordination for a unified strength. Combined with continuous regular and even breathing, the four limbs will be natural, carefree, and comfortable in form and gesture.

Liang Zhen Pu Eight Diagram Palm

SONG 2

First pile up the rear elbow to have the elbow hiding heart,
Then the hand turns and drops to follow forward.
Follow the anterior elbow with a holding power,
The anterior hand and posterior hand in a group of spirits.

Annotation: "Pile up the elbow" means to flex and fold the rear arm inward with the elbow close to the chest. "The hand turns and drops" means that both the hands press and drop toward the center of the circle simultaneously from the previous upward palms position. "A holding power" and "a group of spirits" refers to the sinking of the shoulders and elbows, and the two arms holding inward simultaneously like embracing an object with the whole body, so that the other parts of the body can be considered as a group of spirits or forces.

This formula puts forth the requirements for both the hands and arms. In the practice of Eight Diagram Palm, first, the arms should extend straight with the palms upward. The rear hand piles up (or braces up) the front elbow to protect the chest and hypochondrium (rib area), this is referred to as "elbow covering the heart." The posterior (rear) hand follows the anterior (forward) hand to stop below and several inches from the elbow joint of the anterior arm. The fingers of both hands push upward and the wrists drop downward, and this naturally facilitates the arms in holding as if embracing an object. The hands are distinguished into the posterior and anterior hands, however, during circle walking or combat, the hands will change simultaneously with the change of the footwork. That is, the anterior hand changes to the posterior hand while the posterior hand changes to the anterior hand. The hands take care of each other and are free in penetration and protection. Actually, the penetration is protection and the protection is penetration since the anterior hand is the posterior hand and the posterior hand is the anterior hand. This relates to the theory of change in Yin and Yang. Therefore, the hands "in a group of spirits" means that both the hands act in a coordinated harmony, externally and internally, for launching with whole body power. That is, "hand follows the foot to open."

Formulae

SONG 3

Walk forward with curved steps and straight foot,
Just as in pushing millstones.
Flex the knee, follow the hip, and the waist turns the foot,
Eyes watch three aspects without wobbling the body.

Annotation: This formula puts forth the requirements for the parts below the waist and hip. In circle walking, it is necessary to walk in a straight way with the lateral foot moving slightly inward. In this way, by walking forward, one will naturally walk in a circle. Because the movement always moves around the center of the circle, it resembles pushing a millstone. Eight Diagram Palm is often practiced by walking a circle with a tree as the center. But, in the walking, it is necessary to flex the knee and sink the gravity from above the waist to the hip and then sink it to the knee and foot for the purpose of greater stability. When sinking the gravity, turn the waist as much as possible toward the center. This forms the gesture of "four parade steps and four oblique-angle hands." Due to the flexed knee and sinking hip, the feet can discriminate in the anterior and posterior; and the false and true. The anterior foot extends forward like walking in water. The lower the gravity sinks, the more stable the body will be, therefore, one should sink the gravity of the body as much as possible. Furthermore, it is necessary to close the knees and lower the hip in order to be nimble in the upper body and stable in the lower body, so that the eyes can watch various directions and are free for observation without the mind and vision being diminished by wobbly instability.

Liang Zhen Pu Eight Diagram Palm

SONG 4

To arrive at the target in a straight motion is not special,
Fluidly circling left and right is preferable.
The left changes to the right and the right changes to the left,
In withdrawing the body and reversing the steps one will find an opening.

Annotation: In the practice of Eight Diagram Palm, it is not enough to know one method of approach. It is necessary to practice on both the left and right sides. Therefore, the circles must be clockwise with counter-clockwise turning and vice versa, and the strokes must be interchanged mutually on both sides. During combat, if you only know the combative skills on the left side, you would be defeated completely, all in a fluster, when the opponent uses right sided combative skills. With proficient practice, one can change the gestures freely, naturally and skillfully either for evasion or retreat, whether the power is great or small.

SONG 5

Step, then turn with the hands following,
The rear palm penetrates out and the forward palm withdraws.
Going and coming without warning,
Like an arrow shot from a bow.

Annotation: This song indicates the significance of the combination of hands and feet. There is a proverb in the Chinese martial arts that says: "Bring rebuke on oneself when the hand reaches without being followed by the foot. True mysterious skill results when the hand and foot reach simultaneously." It is a great shortcoming in the attacking skill if the hands are not in close coordination with the feet. Without the synergism of whole body power in hand-foot action, the hand attack would not only lack power if the foot should reach before the hand, but also be extremely risky because "the hands were slow to engage the enemy." When the hand reaches before the foot, although it is possible to attack an opponent, the power may not be strong enough due to the

Formulae

lack of root. In this instance, it is easy to lose both power and posture at the same time and could be a major factor in being defeated. Another proverb regarding close coordination between the hands and feet says: "The hands follow the step to open." This is exactly the meaning of the second sentence in the song. "Going and coming without warning" means that both hands come and go in a manner difficult to anticipate. This action resembles tearing the silk floss. The hand goes out to attack the opponent and comes back to pull the opponent down. Therefore, the hand must extend as quickly and powerfully as the arrow shot from the bow. But there are two details to note in releasing the power:

a) The coming and going of the hands must be accomplished by the turning of the waist;

b) Only eighty or ninety percent of power should be released. The remaining power is retained for other last minute changes with the hands and for releasing the power a second time, if necessary.

SONG 6

Move the fingers and palm forward close to the elbow in penetration,
Posterior shoulder changes to anterior shoulder.
Don't leave space and don't hesitate,
To kick the groin with direct accuracy is a primary consideration.

Annotation: This song is a continuation of the previous song. The previous song requires the coordination of the upper and the lower and the sufficient power and speed of the two hands. This song describes how to penetrate the palm and to coordinate with the feet to ones best advantage. The tips of the fingers must be projected directly toward the opponent in a penetrating palm. The posterior hand is projected forward close to the elbow of the anterior arm while the anterior hand is pulled back to the elbow of the posterior arm by sinking the arm and shoulder. In the alternating penetration of both hands, the anterior and posterior hands mutually change their position. It is important to properly coordinate the footwork in penetrating palm. Specifically, the left foot is anterior when the left hand penetrates, and the right foot is anterior when the right hand penetrates. At the same time, the foot is required to thrust directly into the groin of the opponent. Applying penetrating palm in this manner displays tremendous power and brings the opponent down immediately. Penetrating Palm is one of the most dynamic skills in Eight Diagram Palm and there is a saying: "Even a brave man fears three penetrations." And here, a second saying must be considered: "The elbow does not leave the hand, the hand does not leave the elbow." In this instance, "don't leave space" means "don't stay too far away" from the opponent or "don't be afraid to close in."

SONG 7

When the chest is kept hollow, the Qi will sink,
Hold up the back and sink the shoulders to extend the arm.
Hold the grain duct while Qi reaches the Dantian area,
The head is straightly erected for brilliant spirit.

Annotation: Eight Diagram Palm is an internal boxing skill. Therefore, it is necessary to combine it with breathing techniques and *Qi* guiding skills. In order for *Qi* to sink to the Dantian area (lower abdomen), it is necessary to hollow the chest, so that the breath will sink to the Dantian area naturally. The hollowing of the chest makes it necessary to spread and round the back. In order to keep the root of the shoulders strong they must drop as well. Therefore, the chest can be kept hollow by stretching the back and by sinking the shoulders and the two arms can extend forward by intention. If they are extended by force, the power would lift the arms to float upward. Because the shoulder and elbow sink downward, the chest is hollow and the back is spread, one can use the intention without physical force for guiding the flow of *Qi* to the Dantian area. But, when *Qi* reaches the Dantian area, it is necessary to hold the grain duct (i.e. draw the anus upward like holding stool). This makes it possible to direct *Qi* to flow into the Conception Vessel, through the Point Huiyin (CV1) and into the Governor Vessel, then to ascend directly to the vertex and to reach Pt. Baihui (GV20), and then to descend through Pt. Renzhong (GV26) to Pt. Duiduan (GV27), connecting with Chengjiang (CV24) by the tongue, and finally descending through the Conception Vessel to the Dantian area. In this manner, *Qi* flows

Formulae

continuously in the whole body. When one meridian is open, a hundred meridians can be open. The spirit[2] would be naturally vigorous and the whole body relaxed. Long-term practice can produce a kind of internal energy (real *Qi*), which can be directed by the intention. In combat, it is possible to "have intention connecting with *Qi* and have *Qi* connecting with force" for displaying infinite power and remaining undefeated.

SONG 8

Do not sway the body when moving,
All relies upon interchange below the knees.
The low stance is controlled by lowering the hips and knees,
In the middle stance one should also lower the legs and waist.

Annotation: There are two explanations of the three parts: a) It refers to the stance for the practice of boxing, the upper part refers to the high stance, the middle part refers to the middle stance and the lower part refers to the lower stance. b) The upper part refers to the hands and arms, the middle part refers to the body trunk, waist and hips, and the lower part refers to the thighs and legs. Eight Diagram Palm overcomes its opponents primarily by turning and circle walking with the footwork, therefore it is mandatory that the legs are highly trained. In circle walking the upper body should not sway and the posture should not bob up and down. In order to avoid this bobbing action, it is necessary to sit the waist and hips downward to sink the root to the legs. Therefore, it is necessary that both legs be flexed and the knees held close. Judging from this description, the circle walking in Eight Diagram Palm is accomplished by properly alternating movement of the two legs below the knees, i.e. "interchange below the knees." By long-term practice in this way, the lower part would be naturally stable, the upper body would not sway and the practitioner can walk the circle freely to understand the axiom "suitable to be still and unsuitable to move in the upper part." The posture and stance in walking the circle can be divided into three levels of performance. The highest level of performance walks in the lowest stance, with the knees and hips at the same level in walking the circle. This kind of training requires a lot of practice time and is very tiring, but the skill can be enhanced greatly in short order. However, it is suitable for most of the practitioners to walk with the middle stance. In walking the circle, it is also required to sink the waist downward. After the waist and the hips sit downward, the legs are developed properly and the power in the thighs is increased so that the whole body is stable and powerful.

SONG 9

Close the lips and mouth with the tongue touching the palate,
All respiration goes through the nose.
When force reaches its peak, release it by speaking "Hun" and "Haa,"
For obtaining the combination of whole energy.

Annotation: Song 7 explains how to sink Qi into the Dantian area with the combination of guiding, inhalation and exhalation skills. Song 9 explains the breathing technique in the power releasing method. The cultivation of Qi must be accomplished through breathing and by closing the lips and rolling the tongue upward to touch the palate. Thus, breathing is conducted through the nose, which allows the breathing to be deep, long, even and thready. Breathing through the mouth renders the breathing gruff and hurried and is not as hygienic. Besides, there are two other advantages when the tongue touches the palate. It produces saliva inside the mouth and prevents dry mouth, dry tongue and dry throat during practice and combat. It also can increase the gastric juice and enhance digestive function when the saliva is swallowed into the abdomen.

There are two kinds of respiration, one is natural respiration and the other is deep respiration. Internal boxing emphasizes the natural respiration. This method inhales fresh air into the Dantian area and then exhales the turbid Qi out in expiration. It is necessary to learn natural respiration in working the breathing skill and $Qigong$, i.e. sink Qi into the Dantian area. By long-term practice, Qi can be accumulated progressively inside the Dantian area. When the skill is perfected, Qi will naturally flow downward, pass through Pt. Huiyin (CV1), and then ascend along the Governor Vessel to Pt. Baihui (GV20) on the vertex, and

Formulae

finally descend along the Conception Vessel and return to the Dantian area. (It is called Heavenly Circulation (*Zhou Tian*) in *Qigong*.) Then, by the tongue touching the palate, *Qi* can flow to the four limbs and all body parts. This dynamic is called "Consolidating all the Body Forces" with breathing techniques or, in Chinese martial arts terminology, "internal energy" or "whole energy." All internal boxing styles emphasize the training and cultivation of this kind of *Qi*. Only through constant practice of this method, can the real goals be attained. The body will be strengthened and the power will seem inexhaustible in combat. To store energy, *Qi* must be guided into the Dantian area. In releasing energy, it is projected through the four limbs, with explosive power, to immediately strike the enemy down. To develop releasing power, it is advisable to speak "Hnn" with a twang and "Haa" with an oral sound for maximizing one's own expression of power by shocking the opponent to momentarily decrease his strength thereby affording an opportunity for victory.

The Chinese martial artists of previous generations used to often say: "Develop tendons, bones and skins externally, cultivate a mouthful of *Qi* internally." They strongly emphasize the cultivation of *Qi* and, therefore, handed down the following formula for cultivation of *Qi*:

> *Clench the teeth and don't open the mouth,*
> *Power cannot come if the mouth opens to exhale Qi.*
> *Understand that Qi should always stay in abdomen,*
> *Do not let Qi rise to the chest when fighting.*
> *Lightly rotating and turning the body,*
> *Thoroughly trains the tendons and bones for a strong structure.*
> *Practice in this manner always,*
> *The body constitution would be solidly stronger than iron.*

Liang Zhen Pu Eight Diagram Palm

SONG 10

Stretch the palm and make the Hukou (Tiger's Mouth) round,
With middle finger and ring finger apart.
First poke and then strike with the wrist bone,
Relax the shoulders and lengthen the waist to penetrate with the steps.

Annotation: This song emphasizes the palm form and method. In the practice of Eight Diagram, it is required to stretch *Hukou* (the part between the thumb and the index finger) round. Thus, the power can be forced to reach the tips of the fingers. No matter standing palm, prone palm, supine palm or slapping palm, it is required to slightly flex the thumb, extend the index and middle fingers straight, and join the ring and small fingers for rounding the palm in a hollow. Pt. Zhongxian on the middle finger and Point Guanxian on the ring finger shouldn't be joined together. Joining these two fingers blocks the free flow of *Qi*. Therefore, when the middle and ring fingers are extended forcefully, they would separate naturally and *Qi* would be easy to flow to the tips of the fingers. The developed finger tips are like iron and steel. In combat, first poke the opponent with the fingers directly, then strike downward with the wrist. At the same time, relax the shoulders and the waist, drop the gravity in the arms for the power of the whole body to pour into the wrist. This then is the way to defeat the enemy with the palm method.

Formulae

SONG 11

Advance with knees close and retreat with knees open,
When changing the palms and steps, lower the body .
Advance or retreat in accordance with the circumstance,
Skillfully arrange the position of the waist and legs.

Annotation: In Eight Diagram Palm, the posture should change and the steps advance with the knees close together like in *kou bu*, so the knees look like they aren't changing even when they are. When the body wants to turn in retreat it is necessary to separate the steps first. In this way, the body can turn actively and nimbly. This is the precise purpose of the *kou bu* and the *bai bu*. Secondly, it is necessary to lower the body slightly in the changing of the palm and posture for stability and nimble turning of the lower part. Generally, all the movements must be governed by the hips and waist. Therefore, regardless of the particular form in advancing or retreating, whatever the change of strokes and postures, whether high postures or lower postures, all are coordinated by the turning of the hips and waist. Consequently, only when the waist and legs are arranged properly is everything else possible.

SONG 12

This palm is quite different from others,
There are skills in advancing steps and lifting the foot.
First move the rear foot in retreat,
Step apart from the center when moving to the side.

Annotation: The most significant characteristics of Eight Diagram Palm emphasize the footwork. The footwork belongs to one of the eight reverses. In combat, it is required to advance with the anterior foot first in the forward attack, in other words, lift the anterior foot away from the ground a little bit and then push off the posterior foot forcefully

Liang Zhen Pu Eight Diagram Palm

then follow it immediately (following step). This takes advantage of the time and the reflex force when the posterior foot suddenly propels one forward from the ground. In terms of the power, the stamping power (root power) of the posterior foot is applied, so that the whole body power can be employed. Therefore, it is said that "it needs this technique to move the anterior foot first." It is required to retreat the posterior foot first while retreating backward, that is, lift the posterior foot away from the ground first and then stamp[3] the anterior foot backward. In terms of the eight diagrams, it is called "the half step advance" or "the half step following." Used in conjunction with whole body power, it is unbeatable. Stepping apart from the center means that when attacked directly in front, a head-on confrontation with the enemy must be avoided. With the bodywork (lateral body method) and footwork (advancing laterally), I can avoid the attack from the enemy and at the same time completely waste his power by drawing him to an empty position. Due to inertia, the enemy's body still moves forward and forfeits his root, so that the enemy loses stability. In side stepping the enemy I can attack him and defeat him before he can regain stability.

SONG 13

This palm is quite different from others,
The hand moves after the shoulder attacks.
First move backward before extension,
Inhaling completely before exhaling, power will be abundant.

Annotation: This song refers to the differences with other boxing arts. That is, before the release of power, it is necessary to first store up power and so is it advisable to release power only after it is fully stored up. This kind of power would be more forceful than the power released without storing it up. When the power is stored up, it is necessary to coordinate it with the natural breath. Thus, the released power would manifest suddenly like a powerful explosion. It is especially necessary to pay attention to the fact that the accumulation and release of the power must originate in the mind (intention), that is, store up the power in the root section and when it is stored up, release it with a jolt. Therefore, it is said that "the hand moves after the shoulder attacks, move backward before extension." This method for storing up and releasing power is found in all internal boxing methods.

Formulae

SONG 14

This palm is quite different from others,
Force is mutually connected between anterior palm and posterior palm.
First move the root when planning to use the tip,
No techniques can be overlooked.

Annotation: This song explains how both hands work in coordination and where the power is released. It is necessary to use whole body power in extending the palm. It has been mentioned already in Song 11 that the root is the foot, and the power originating from the leg is controlled by the waist and manifests in the fingers. Whole body power must release from the root section. This is why it is said to move the root first while planning to use the tip. "The power is mutually connected in both hands" refers to a kind of synergistic force and a separating force. Thus, it is possible for the anterior hand to release more forceful power when the posterior hand draws backward to have pulling power. This is the so-called "going and coming without any warning" mentioned in Song 5. Both in training and combat, this method is very important and cannot be neglected. It must be executed accurately, forcefully and with stability.

SONG 15

This palm is quite different from others,
First feint to the east before attacking the west.
Know how to point to the upper and strike the lower,
Great skill is to roll pearls upward.

Annotation: It is necessary for the practitioners of Eight Diagram Palm to understand the military art which includes many special strategies and tactics, such as feint to the east while attacking the west,

Liang Zhen Pu Eight Diagram Palm

create something out of nothing, seizing that which is within easy reach, let the enemy go in order to catch him, catch fish in troubled water, befriend the distant enemy while attacking the nearer one, feign madness without becoming insane, make a guest to be the host, lure the tiger out of the mountains, evasion is the best plan, etc. All these strategies and tactics can be used accordingly in combat. In particular, if the tactics of the firm-gentle force, frontal and lateral attack, advance and retreat for attacking and defense, and deception in battle are all applied to make a feint to the east while attacking the west or to point to the upper while hitting the lower, it renders the opponent confused and defenseless. If I "know the enemy and myself, I can fight a hundred battles with no danger of defeat." The so-called "roll pearls upward" means to strike from the ground up; that is, to use the vibrating power of the whole body power. Therefore, it is necessary for the practitioners of Eight Diagram Palm to practice and study "drilling-turning power, twisting-rotating power, shocking-springing power, bursting-exploding power, vibrating-shaking, drilling power" and their methods. These are also employed in other boxing methods.

SONG 16

Those with natural proficient skill still fear the three penetrations,
Not moving to the outside is a waste of time.
He walks outside and I walk inside,
It's not difficult to attack with the extending hand.

Annotation: Applying three successive penetrating palms is a major tactic in Eight Diagram Palm. It is said that even a natural fighter fears the three penetrations and this song refers to some details that one must be aware of to utilize the three penetrating palms. When I continuously penetrate with the palms and change sides toward the enemy, the opponent becomes confused and disoriented, so that I can seize the advantage and defeat him. But, during the palm penetration, the footwork walks on the left and right.

Formulae

SONG 17

It is not a skill to use the palm in only one way,
At least be proficient in four ways.
One crossing and one straight form triangle hands,
It's like embracing a person in my bosom.

Annotation: The third sentence of this song talks about the principle of the handwork and the last sentence talks about the result of the skillful utilization of the handwork. Both the handwork and footwork should be set in a triangle. With one hand across the body and the other hand extended straight, a triangle can be formed in the center from which infinite changes can be created. In combat, I can neutralize the enemy's straightness with my transverseness and can attack the enemy's transverseness with my straightness, thus, even through the changes the triangles are still present. This triangle creates a specific posture the image of which feels as though one were embracing something to their chest. This develops a strong skill to embrace. So that when the enemy is in my bosom, I can manipulate him wantonly, as well as having a reinforced triangle that can keep him out, if that is my desire.

SONG 18

Attack a tall person low and a short person high,
If angling the body and changing steps one can stay calm.
Waist force is required in oblique turning and reverse turning,
Firm force is like steel when rotation reaches its utmost.

Annotation: When the enemy is taller than me, I attack his lower part with my lower posture. If the enemy is shorter than me, I use my advantage to attack him in the upper part with my high posture. Consequently, neither the tall person nor the short person can resist me. No matter how the postures change, it is necessary to take advantage of the enemy's failed attack and defeat him. In the eyes of the enemy I am directly in front of him but, in fact, I will be to his lateral side. That is, I would avoid a head-on fight with the enemy evading laterally then moving in immediately to counter attack. This is the better way to seek victory. The waist is the governor of the whole body, therefore, all the oblique or reverse turning should be accomplished by the movement of the waist. The release of firm force is applied at the furthest reach of the waist rotation.

SONG 19

It's said that the palm method wins from its firmness,
Master Guo used to mention gentleness is hidden inside.
It's secret has been known by some people,
Combination of firmness and gentleness is its advantage.

Annotation: Master Guo, that is Mr. Guo Ji Yuan, was a native of Zhaoyuan County, Shandong Province. There are many styles in his boxing skills, but the nature of the releasing power can be explained in two types: a) the firm power (hard exercise) and b) gentle power (soft exercise). The whole body power is used to attack the opponent in Eight Diagram Palm, to let the opponent feel infinite power. It is often thought that the firm-strong power is used to triumph over the opponent, however, this is not the case. Mr. Guo described: "Eight Diagram Palm is a boxing skill with the combination of firmness and gentleness." Therefore, the practitioners must understand that the combination of firmness and gentleness is essential in all the boxing techniques. Generally speaking, firmness and gentleness are explained often to beginners. When the skills are proficient, it is natural to regulate gentleness and firmness freely. At that moment, it is not possible to distinguish them clearly. The saying "long fist is not long and short fist is not short" specifically refers to this dynamic.

Formulae

SONG 20

Firmness appears first with gentleness hidden inside,
Gentleness comes first with firmness followed.
When he moves his waist and hands by gentleness,
I would suck in with the waist and move stable steps.

Annotation: The boxing skill of mutual support in firmness and gentleness has been explained somewhat in the previous songs. This song further explains the principle of the mutual support of firmness and gentleness. Before we use the firm power, it is necessary to apply stable, soft power. It is called "the gentleness hidden within the firmness." Before the firm power is applied, it is necessary to have the gentle power stored. This is called "the firmness stored within gentleness." Neither attack nor defense is without this principle, especially in combat. When the opponent attacks with gentle power, I can deal with it by firm power. If he uses firm power, I use gentle power to absorb it with the waist and footwork, then attack back and triumph over him. Although firmness and gentleness can change at any time, it's successful change depends upon the assistance of the footwork.

SONG 21

When in the extreme, the body must turn,
Get myself free and move my shadow without leaving a trace.
Deception is carried out in footwork,
The waist must extend first in advance and retreat.

Liang Zhen Pu Eight Diagram Palm

Annotation: The "extreme" refers to the linking movement of two postures. "Get myself free and move my shadow" refers to the bodywork. That Eight Diagram Palm can triumph over all others depends upon the footwork. If the footwork is properly executed, it is possible to do whatever is necessary. But the change of the footwork and numerous changes in the handwork must be coordinated through the waist. This is why it is said: "To bring the steps with the waist, to turn the body with the steps, to change the palm with the body and to turn the steps with the palm by coordination of the upper and the lower."

SONG 22

The spirit in turning the palm is transmitted from the neck bone,
The hand moves before turning the neck.
Extend the neck for releasing power and pull it down for changes,
Like a spiritual dragon linking its head and tail together.

Annotation: To project the image of a bright spirit and acute alertness, it is necessary to hold the neck erect. If the neck is erect, the energy would be transmitted naturally to the vertex, and the spirit would radiate energy. The spinal column is the mainstay of the human body with the cervical vertebrae connecting the head with the rest of the spinal column. Hence, it's role is critical in maintaining the overall posture and if the neck is crooked, the proper posture is impossible. It is necessary for "the eyes to follow the hands to move and the hands to follow the eyes to move." This is why the hand should move before turning the neck. As for "extend neck for releasing power and pull it down for changes," it means that the neck must be relaxed and natural while changing the gestures and storing up the energy. Moving the head and neck upward in releasing the power increases the power that is released. When the skills in the eyes, hands, body, methods and footwork are combined together, it links the head and tail energetically.

Formulae

SONG 23

When striking the opponent with the hand the shoulder is its root,
It is not possible to extend the tip if the arm movement is not from the shoulder.
Advance the forward foot when the enemy wants to advance,
It is futile to advance the back foot.

Annotation: The first three sentences discuss the engaging of the root before applying the tip in combat. This has been explained previously and need not be repeated here. The fourth sentence talks about the necessity to first advance the anterior step, followed by the posterior step. To advance with the posterior step would be too slow and, therefore, in vain.

SONG 24

Strong force is released from tendons and bones,
Firmness from the bones is channeled by the tendons.
The big tendon of the heel connects with the spine and head,
Extend the power by using the follow step.

Annotation: Power is required in the attacking skills. But this kind of power must be whole body power and cannot be ordinary undeveloped power. This power is generated from the bones and is called "firm power." The powerful force generated from the tendons is called gentle power. Both kinds of power are combined together to form whole body power of the mutual support between firmness and gentleness, i.e. the so-called "power with root." The release of this power must start from the heel, passing the thigh, the waist and back and out to the fingers. This powerful force can take down anything.

Liang Zhen Pu Eight Diagram Palm

SONG 25

The eyes reach simultaneously with the hand, waist and leg,
Supported by real heart, real spirit and real force.
Combination of three reals and four reaches,
Enough to defend self and defeat others.

Annotation: Besides the close coordination of the hands, eyes, body, methods and footwork, it is also required in Eight Diagram Palm that "the heart is combined with the mind (spirit), the mind is combined with *Qi* (breath) and *Qi* is combined with the power (force)." This is the three reals and four combinations, i.e. "the combination of the three interior with the exterior produces an entire body." While the eyes are watching the enemy, the hands are sensing the enemy, the mind is analyzing his interior and the whole being is threatening to attack his position whatever it is. Whether attacking or defending, one can handle the situation with ease and win the victory.

SONG 26

Force should be both hard and soft,
Overemphasis on either firmness or gentleness leads to imbalance.
It is true that overly firm objects are easily broken,
Things that are too soft have no power.

Annotation: The firmness and gentleness of the power has been explained in Song 19 and Song 20. This song refers to when a boxer tries to secure victory by stubbornly employing firmness, or to achieve a purely soft win by only gentleness. Boxing skills that stress either firmness or gentleness as a ploy would be unable to prevail over the internal boxing skill where firmness and gentleness are combined. Because the rigid substance is crisp in nature and easy to break and soft substance is weak and easy to wither, the power released must be properly blended in firmness and gentleness, i.e. "to break it with

Formulae

firmness and to absorb it with gentleness." If these key principles are understood, it is possible to master the boxing skills.

SONG 27

We are speaking of hard and soft in balance,
It is not difficult to have mutual dependence between firmness and gentleness.
Gentleness and firmness should be used with the Qian and Kun hands,
To lift heaven and open the ground like the endless surging of waves in the sea.

Annotation: Yin and Yang, true and false, firmness and gentleness, softness and hardness are opposites. These opposites are mutually supporting. Therefore, over-doing or under-doing, which respectively refer to over-firmness, over-hardness, over-truth, over-yang or over-yin, over-softness, over-false and over-gentleness, all lead to defeat. This is why it is said in the previous song: "Overemphasis on either firmness or gentleness leads to imbalance." Consequently, those who research boxing skills must understand that "firmness can correct the excess of gentleness to avoid weakness, gentleness can decrease the excess of the firmness to avoid losing strong power." This is the mutual dependence between firmness and gentleness that allows the complementary aspects to be utilized. In practical application, it is easy to understand the real meaning of true and false, which can change at any time. The anterior hand is true and the posterior hand is false, or vice versa. One hand alone can also be divided into true and false. The two legs can be divided into true and false, the upper part and lower part of the body can be divided into true and false, and all the directions can be divided into true and false. If the principle of true and false is understood it is easy to achieve victory. As for the Qian hand and Kun hand, Qian means the heaven (representing yang-firmness) and Kun means the earth (representing yin-gentleness). In other words, one hand is truth and the other hand is false. The hands can be used alternating the left and right to attack high and low, with the power of surging waves.

SONG 28

It is right method that I am in gentleness and he is in firmness,
It is also a good method that I am in firmness and he is in gentleness.
When firmness and gentleness meet, victory is decided through superior body method,
Strict footwork can solve the dispute.

Annotation: When the opponent attacks me with a firm force, I can defend myself by footwork and gentle force to avoid the firm attack of the opponent. If I attack the opponent with firm force, the opponent can also avoid my attack with gentle force. If, however, I meet a strong opponent, it is hard to say who will win. Under this situation, I must deal with the opponent with the bodywork (waist). On the other hand, bodywork must rely upon the footwork. Generally, when firmness and gentleness meet, it is necessary to deal with the opponent by the bodywork and footwork for the victory. It means that "if opportunity and advantage are not present, it is necessary to rely upon the waist and legs."

SONG 29

First lift the waist in movement of footwork,
Mystery would appear in proper retraction.
If the waist doesn't move when the foot needs to move,
Opportunity would be lost by staggered steps.

Annotation: Previously, the footwork has been explained. Now, some details in moving the steps are presented. The waist and hips are the governor of the whole body, therefore, every movement must be at the command of the waist and hips. That is to say, the waist is the axis

Formulae

to move the four limbs. In this case, "to lift the waist" means to rotate the waist slightly before moving the step in walking the circle. "Retraction" here means to slightly retract the hip. That is, both the hips should alternate in the true and false. If the left foot needs to lift, the weight should be shifted to the right hip with a slight lifting of the left hip. If the right foot needs to lift, the weight should be shifted to the left hip with a slight lifting of the right hip. In this way, the alternating footwork can be natural, light, nimble and active. Mr. Liang Zhen Pu used to say: "Lift without showing it, just lift with the mind." In summary, to move the step without moving the waist would result in stiff movement and staggering steps. In combat, the staggering would provide the enemy an opportunity, therefore, is highly prohibited.

SONG 30

Don't over extend the steps in turning the body and changing gestures,
Don't be flustered while sweeping ground to move.
Perceiving invading strikes, only extend an arm,
Steadily, softly and firmly as a smart girl threading a needle.

Annotation: When it is necessary to change gesture and stroke, one needs to use small steps. It is inadvisable to apply big steps. Small steps allow nimble, rapid rotation and change and can release a quick striking force that none can dodge. While in combat, it is necessary to have a calm mind and stable steps without any haste in observing the attack; merely extend the arm to deal with it. The last sentence means that the needle is hard, the thread is soft and the eye of the needle is small. The person who threads the needle's eye must be calm in mind and steady in hands to work with the tiny needle and soft thread. Only in this way can the thread be put through the eye of the needle. It means that it is necessary to have keen observation, calm mind and skillful hands.

Liang Zhen Pu Eight Diagram Palm

SONG 31

No need to worry when he takes a sharp weapon,
Attacking with his sword toward my body from far away.
Escape by voicing "Hun" and "Haa" after spotting his strokes,
It is an excellent phrase that "evil never can triumph over righteousness."

Annotation: In combat, success depends first on courage and second on skill. Therefore, there is a saying: "When one man is willing to risk his life, he can hold out against ten thousand." So, it is necessary to boost one's courage. The bolstered courage can produce a calm mind and a calm mind allows for keen observation and keen observation can ensure quick striking. In combat, no matter what sharp weapons he uses, even if he chops with his sword near my body, I must be calm in dealing with it, spotting the invading gestures and extending the arm to ward it off. Then by using "Hun" and "Haa" loudly to shock him, the enemy, momentarily frightened, loses his advantage and I can seize the opportunity to defeat him. So, when the opponent is fearful enough to attempt to draw extra advantage in weapon or circumstance, this evil can be countered and overcome with courage and a" spirit cry."

SONG 32

Defense in close combat seems difficult,
Especially when a sharp fish-intestine sword is present.
Which is easy to draw like taking an object from a pocket,
Mystery is hidden while pointing at the mountain for making a millstone.

Annotation: The fish-intestine sword which was said to be manufactured by Ou Yan-zi in the Spring-Autumn Period, has an extremely sharp blade. Prince Wu in the Wu State sent an assassin to

Formulae

assassinate and overthrow King Liao with this sword hidden inside the fish's belly. This is how the sword was named. This song is a continuation of the previous song. It is emphasized again that the mind must be calm in combat with the enemy, to wait for the movement with calmness, even though there is a sharp fish-intestine sword involved. Although calm and stable in the mind and able to spot the invading gestures, the enemy also has a sharp weapon, therefore, using the tactics of "making a feint to the east while attacking in the west" will puzzle the enemy and draw him in, providing an opportunity to attack and win the victory.

SONG 33

It is difficult to resist the force of many attackers single handed,
But to offset a thousand pound force with skill is not a bother.
Finger force can be used instead of the whole hand,
Even a strong ox fears the bow turning power.

Annotation: Combating many attackers alone is difficult and it is necessary to win by strategy. The small scale can weigh a thousand pound object by turning on its pivot. In combat with many attackers, it is necessary to use the tactics of "making a feint to the east while attacking in the west" and of "attacking the weak point after evading the real strike" with a calm mind and bolstered courage. This is crucial in a situation where one person combats many attackers. In combat against a single enemy, it is also sometimes necessary to understand how to take advantage of the other person's force. For example, the ox is big in body and very strong in it's power, but if it's horn is turned, it is possible to throw the ox down. Therefore, it is possible to conquer the opponent just by an intelligent move.

Liang Zhen Pu Eight Diagram Palm

SONG 34

If extending the hand forward without seeing the palm,
Without oilish pine tree shining his body.
Focus the eyes widely and stare carefully,
Play lower postures for securing miracles.

Annotation: Torches of pitchy pine twigs were ignited for luminance during night battles in ancient times. This song tells how to deal with the situation in which enemies are encountered in the dark night without lanterns or light. The best way is to use a lower stance so that it is easier to see the opponent clearly and it is convenient to carry out the skills and tactics.

SONG 35

In icy weather, snowy ground and slippery, rainy days,
Carefully step the forward foot flat in kou bu as always.
It is highly prohibited to pivot the foot on the ground,
This is the best method to avoid stumbling in uneven terrain.

Annotation: This song discusses how to deal with the situation if the enemy is confronted on rainy or snowy days when it is difficult to walk on the slippery ground. The song emphasizes the footwork, that is, step the forward foot in kou bu as usual, paying special attention to setting the foot down flat without pivoting. In this way, the forward foot steps down solidly contacting as large an area as possible (full size of the foot) so that it would be less likely to slip forward. Stepping transversely with the anterior foot must coincide with the hips and knees in a stable root so that the entire foot steps down at once and does not slip forward or backward. This provides a stable stance for advancing, retreating and turning. It is highly prohibited to step the foot straight forward. Straight

Formulae

steps touch the ground in a small area (i.e. the heel) and, therefore, it is easy to slip forward, resulting in a backward fall. In turning the body for changing gestures and postures, it is highly prohibited to have a screw-like turning with the heel or ball, because this pivot point is too small in the turning of the body and therefore, not stable enough to ensure against falling. It is necessary to lift the foot completely away from the ground and then either *kou* or *bai* the step accordingly. After the foot steps on the ground completely, the body gravity can be shifted and the other foot can be lifted for the change of the posture. Consequently, it is possible to stand with stability without ever losing balance. It is necessary to pay close attention to the terrain and whether or not there are any obstructions on the ground. This is also very important to enable one to stand as stable as Mount Taishan.

SONG 36

It is important to have spirit in application,
Brilliant spirit enables the ears and eyes to be more intensified.
Even if his hands fly like a sparrow,
I can sense ants and bugs singing like roaring from tiger and dragon.

Annotation: While in combat, the most important thing is to concentrate the mind and have a calm mind and stable spirit for the whirling spiritual energy, which would enable the ears to hear more clearly and the eyes to see more clearly. No matter how violent and quick the enemy is, the principle of waiting for the movement in the calm stillness is vital. In this way one can sense every movement of the enemy, hearing the chirping of the ants and bugs like the roaring from a tiger or dragon. This describes the quick response of the sensory organs.

Liang Zhen Pu Eight Diagram Palm

SONG VERSE

Palm and fist methods discussed on mountains,
Passed down for long time and maybe forgotten.
Although thirty-six songs I sing,
Every sentence implies real meaning.

Annotation: The above-mentioned thirty-six songs were studied in the mountains by Master Dong Hai Chuan. He passed down his experiences with the training methods of the Eight Diagram Palm and noteworthy points to be mindful of in avoiding mistakes and how to combine them with breathing methods. Every word and sentence of these songs has profound implications which contain the principles of the Eight Diagram Palm and hold the intricate mystery for the practice of the Eight Diagram Palm. Therefore, all students must memorize these songs. Only by having these songs at your immediate access is it possible to use them freely and appreciate the many insights and attain real skills after long-time practice.

ESSENTIAL FORMULAE OF FORTY-EIGHT METHODS AND THEIR ANNOTATIONS

1) Body Method

Hand and foot methods must follow each other,
Power will be a little if the foot steps down after the hand reaches out.
Without the waist even the hand and foot reaching out together lacks power,
It's difficult to retreat if going slowly.

Annotation: The internal boxing methods require that the hand, eyes, body, method and steps be in close coordination for generating whole body power for striking the enemy. Whole body power depends upon the foot as its root, controlled by the waist for the coordination of the interior and exterior and the upper and lower to strike the enemy to the ground. If the hand has already punched the enemy's body and the foot has not yet thrust into the groin of the opponent, then the power applied is only the local power of the hand, not whole body power. Even if the hand and foot can coordinate, without any assistance from the waist power, the power applied is still only the local power of the hand and foot and will not produce the strongest effect. Further, lack of close coordination between the hand, foot and waist, would slow the movement in advance and retreat as well as impede turning, which can lead to one's defeat. Therefore, it is mandatory that the eyes, body, hand, method and steps are closely coordinated. It is also required that the heart should be combined with the intention, the intention with Qi, and Qi with the force of action so that internal harmony will coordinate with the upper and the lower and the interior with the exterior to create whole body power, which is able to strengthen the body, prevent illness and prolong life, as well as guarantee victory in combat.

Liang Zhen Pu Eight Diagram Palm

2) Surveying Method

First survey around in battle with enemy,
Evade before advancing steps.
Retreat for surveying and understanding changes,
To wait at ease for fatigued enemy can produce great power.

Annotation: First of all, regardless of how many enemies there are, it is necessary to observe the enemy's force and estimate the enemy's weak points. It is said that it is important to estimate correctly your own strength as well as that of your enemy, so that even in hundreds of battles there will be no defeat. Therefore, before the enemy's strength is known, it is inadvisable to advance rashly. It is always wise to consider the value of evasion. This does not mean fear of the opponent's abilities but rather that by evading one is able to appraise the opponent's situation so as to avoid the powerful position, attack the weak point, and thereby secure victory. The skillful and experienced fighter can either advance or retreat. If one is only able to advance and does not know how to use retreat or vice versa, he is unlikely to be successful in battle and will most likely be defeated.

When your own weakness is known, the strategy of evasion can cover your weak point, it buys time to search for opportunity in the retreating steps. Initially, the opponent has the advantage, however, when his attack reveals his weak point, I can seize the moment to defeat him. This is the method to survey the situation, know the options and then conquer him with my remaining strength. In the situation of waiting at ease for a fatigued enemy, a small force is usually very effective.

Formulae

3) Stepping Method

Move the root before moving the tip,
Fast hands are not as good as following with a half step.
Walk a half step in advance and retreat,
Calmly evade strokes and conquer the opponent.

Annotation: This formula refers to the importance of the foot method. How to first engage the root when the tip is to be applied has been explained in the previous songs, but the concept of tip and root is relative. In terms of the lower section, the foot is the tip and the hip is the root. In terms of the whole body, the hands and head are the tip and the waist and hips are the middle joints and the legs and feet are the root. Therefore, the power should be released from the foot to the waist and to the hand. In terms of the hands, it means that the waist supports the arm and the elbow supports the palm. The Eight Diagram Palm strikes the opponent with a whole body power, destroying his root and throwing him far away and down. But, regardless of how smart and fast your hands are, it is necessary to have coordinated footwork. The footwork in Eight Diagram Palm is unique in Chinese martial arts and requires only a half step to change gestures and strokes in advancing, retreating and turning. This step can be used even in attacking and evading the opponent. Therefore, it is necessary to remember "first the half step" or "to follow with the half step." When practiced to perfection, it is very easy to safeguard yourself and conquer the enemy.

4) Walking Method

Attacking power originates from bent legs,
Two hands follow the steps to change.
Block high, brush low, and shield across,
Pushing, uplifting, carrying, and leading never leave the chest.

Liang Zhen Pu Eight Diagram Palm

Annotation: The skills of the Eight Diagram Palm are derived from circle-walking. This kind of circle-walking by stepping to the left with the right foot and turning the upper body to the right and by stepping to the right with the left foot and turning the upper body to the left is the way the hands change with the steps. There is a saying in the art of war that "of the thirty-six plans, evasion is the best," this is a functional strategy in the walking method of Eight Diagram Palm. Strategically, it means that walking is not only walking, but circling with the enemy as well. In fact, the skills of whole body power and changing of the hands are gradually acquired from circle walking. The hands will change continuously with turning and walking. Therefore, it is said that "the hands follow the steps to change." When the handwork, footwork and bodywork are closely coordinated, the skills can be perfected. In combat, it is necessary to bring all skills and abilities into full play against the opponent and protect yourself in all directions by pushing, pulling, seizing and controlling. But, the most fundamental method relies upon the application of the mind and intention. That is, when the state of "the mind followed by the movements" is manifested, invincibility is possible in every battle.

5) Linking Step Method

It takes a long time to link steps,
In use, the hand should be simple and natural.
Emptiness in hand touching hand and turning body,
Opportunity appears just in front of the skillful master.

Annotation: The footwork mentioned in this formula, such as the ring-chained step, advancing step, retreating step and backing step, has its own magic effect. It is performed freely and according to what is appropriate without strictly adhering to any set form. A set form would only hinder its applications in combat. It is same for the handwork. There are no inflexible rules which restrict the manner in which it must be applied. It is necessary to apply the methods freely according to the individual circumstance. All techniques are interchangeable. Effectiveness in practical application determines what is appropriate. In combat, I may simply turn and move away after touching the hand of

Formulae

the opponent. This is a ploy to lure the enemy, to bait him into striking, then I simply turn my body to evade his strike. Because the touching hand is empty, the opponent's body will tend to fall forward when he misses his strike, so that he loses his posture in the lower body and pulls out his root, and thereby loses stability. At this moment, I can turn the body again and strike him while he is off balance. Surely, he will fall down. Therefore, it is said that "opportunity appears just in front of the skillful master."

6) Step Hoarding Method

Steps cannot hoard equally on the same line,
It is proper to be in false power in anterior and in real power in posterior.
If standing on the same line and moving backward and forward,
Even great chance will be lost because of shortness in the waist.

Annotations: This formula addresses the stance. There is no definite form for holding the stance in walking and turning. In the changes of the gestures and strokes, there is occasional stops in the footwork for a brief period of time, but just for an instant. This is referred to as the hoarded steps. In combat, the correct stance is such that both feet cannot stand on the same line and rather must stand with one foot in front with false force and the other in back with real force. If the two feet stand on the same line, it is easy to push the body backward or pull it forward, as well as lead to awkward and clumsy movements in advancing, retreating and turning, which results in lack of distinction in the real and false force in the feet. This can lead to defeat. The Eight Diagram Palm requires distinctive false and real forces. The feet must stand with the false force in one foot and the real force in the other foot, allowing nimble and free advancing and retreating appropriate for both attack and defense. Otherwise, even if the opponent gives you an opportunity, you will probably not be able to use it.

7) Hand Method

Uneven balance will be followed by double weightedness and stagnation,
Hard on the exterior and soft in the interior like the force of a whipping spear.
Pushing a transverse attack and hooking an inward attack my body will be under control,
Only then can the hand withdraw with the waist following.

Annotation: The methods of the hands and feet are similar. Regardless of hand or foot, it is inadvisable to be double weighted, because double weightedness is stagnant and clumsy. It is better to be single weighted, i.e. one substantial and one insubstantial. Further, in the application of the hand method, it is also required to be hard on the exterior and soft in the interior, like the picking power in the spear head with the intention of penetrating. When the enemy's hand comes in transversely, I push it away. When the enemies hand attacks straight in, I hook it. Generally, this will guide the opponent's power and divert his force, causing the opponent to lose his balance and to miss his strike while my body remains stable. This is the best way to win the victory. Therefore, no matter how fiercely and rapidly the opponent attacks, my way to victory is to hollow the chest and draw the opponent in with the hand with the waist and abdomen following.

8) Power Method

People talk about cold, springing, crisp, rapid and hard power,
I say cold and springing power is very ordinary.
There is no difference between crisp and hard power,
Power release depends upon combination of mind and force.

Formulae

Annotation: All boxing methods talk about the qualities of cold, springing, rapid, crisp and hard power. The practitioners of Eight Diagram Palm say that the cold (sudden) power and rapid power together form the springing power. Therefore, the cold and rapid powers are related. The crisp power and hard power look a little different but, in fact, inside the two powers cannot be separated. The crisp power does not mean its not hard, but we cannot say that they are different. The Eight Diagram Palm requires whole body power. By moving *Qi* with the mind and moving the body with *Qi*, the power starts from the Dantian area and descends to Pt. Yongquan (K1) in the sole, then ascends to the leg, waist and back, and finally issuing out from the hand. In this way, the application of the force relies upon intention and the mind.

9) Power Storing Method

If one only knows how to use power without knowing how to store power,
Power goes just like an arrow leaving its bow.
Which is not only useless but also harmful,
Either leading to defeat or to injury of the body.

Annotation: The power should not all be released at once as it is necessary to always reserve some power. If every bit of power is released like shooting an arrow that doesn't return, it is very easy to be at risk. Therefore, the effort is not only wasted but possibly harmful and may lead to defeat. When I punch the opponent, I use his inertia when he misses his strike and loses his balance. Therefore, at the same time I must be sure of my punch to the opponent, leaving no chance to be countered. Those who release all the power at once do not know the whole body power and do not understand the principle of the false and real force. How can they help but be injured and defeated in combat?

10) Power Increasing Method

His root has already been broken when he is struck by power,
Surely he will not escape if power is applied again.
In the moment, steps should be charged forward,
With long arm and long waist handed in simultaneously.

Annotation: In the situation when the opponent's power is pulled away by me or his root is moved in releasing power, if I change the gestures and strokes (reposition) to follow up and punch him again, he can also adjust his posture to a stable stance to deal with me. Therefore, before the opponent can regain stability and before he regathers his power, I can use my reserve power to attack the opponent continuously and end the fight. But when I use my reserve power, I must advance my steps forward, relax my waist and shoulders, and lower my body further.

11) People Vanquishing Method

No need to boast of rapidness beating slowness,
Strong controlling weak is not special.
Best is to be superior in technique,
With center equilibrium, power is not issued in vain.

Annotation: This formula implies that the students must practice painstakingly. Only when you have more skill than the others, are you able to do whatever you want.

Formulae

12) Victory Method

When his power is as heavy as a thousand pound weight and as quick as a shuttle,
Evade his strong attack by following it.
Among thousands of people, only three to five can be close,
It's not difficult to protect just by extending the hand and foot slightly.

Annotation: The above formula says that it is not necessary to win the battle with power. It refers to the method of striking the weak spot by evading the strong. In combat, no matter how fast the hand is and how powerful the strike is, I persist in the method of conquering the movement with stillness and waiting at ease for the fatigued enemy and observing his strokes. Then I follow his powerful strike to alter the direction of his power so that he will miss his strike and lose his posture. When the direction of the opponent's force is being controlled, victory is certain if the footwork is coordinated. Secondly, when I deal with several people at one time, I should be calm and persist in the method of dealing with the various changes by no special change in my strategy. Although there are many enemies around me, only three to five of them can be near me. Therefore, I must observe their skills carefully and find out the weak one and attack him. So, it is said that "it's not difficult to protect just by extending hand and foot slightly."

13) Application Method

Strike the tall low and the short high,
Strike fat at an angle, no need to waiver.
Rely on guiding methods when facing thin and tall people,
Look up and down without any power when meeting an old man.

Liang Zhen Pu Eight Diagram Palm

Annotation: The Eight Diagram Palm is also called the Eight Reverse Palm. This formula talks about how to apply the method of the Eight Reverse Palm with different types of opponents. For one who is taller than me, I can attack his lower body with the low gesture and force him to pay attention to the lower part, so that he is unable to take advantage of his height and reach. For one who is shorter than me, I can attack his head with the high gesture, so that he cannot carry out his skills at lower level attack. For a fat person, I avoid his front and attack his side or back, because the fat body is slow and difficult to turn and their abilities will be lost in turning. For one who is thin and tall, I use the method of seizing his body, so that he will lose the ability because of the body being controlled and thrown. When confronting weak and aged people, just stare at them and they will be confused and scared. Therefore, you can prevail without moving the hand or foot. Generally speaking, no matter what your opponent looks like, you can win by employing the walking, turning and rotating skills of the Eight Diagram Palm.

14) Blocking Method

Three junctures extend and flex in the hand and leg,
There are three junctures in one hand while the foot straightens and bends.
Shoulders, elbows, wrists, hips and knees can be used,
Move the neck downward, empty the chest with footwork guiding the body.

Annotation: The three junctures in the arm refer to the shoulder, elbow and wrist, and the three junctures in the leg refer to the hip, knee and ankle. In combat, it is required to close the upper three junctures, while the three junctures of the lower part should be flexed and extended for circle walking and turning. This is the blocking method of the whole body. The application of all three junctures must be decided by the straight and curved movement in the steps. Although the hands are used depending upon the footwork, the proper effect will only take place through the coordination of the bodywork.

Formulae

15) Connecting Method

Miscellaneous variation in a big mess,
Mixed with long fist and short strike.
If the quicker you are, the slower I am,
Both Gods and devils would praise when I fight.

Annotation: In Chinese martial arts, there is a wide variety of boxing skills, each having their strong points. When these skills are applied, the fist strikes and the leg kicks in every direction like wind in a storm. At that time, I can still persist in the principle of wait in stillness for movement and to calmly observe the attacking method of the opponent. No need to strive even for a moment for a courageous reputation. Therefore, it is said that "the quicker you are, the slower I am." When I want to release my power, I would take advantage of his weak point to strike him with whole body power. Surely, he will be defeated under my powerful attack. Therefore, it is said that "even Gods and devils will praise when I fight."

16) Dissolving Method

Don't boast about many capture skills,
When two hands grab one, power is stuck.
Even his skillful capture would be afraid of being pushed over head,
Power cannot be resisted if the nose and eyes are pierced.

Annotation: The Eight Diagram Palm does not require the capture method in combat. If someone grabs you, you just push the hands over the head, which can eliminate his power and dissolve his ability. Then, if I punch his nose with my hand and pierce his eyes with my fingers to disturb him, his capture skill will be completely useless.

17) Method of Accepting the Single to Support the Double

Don't say two hands have strong weapons,
It's real skill to have one coming and other going.
When the right hand is blocked, the left will be useless,
No power will appear if two hands come at the same time.

Annotation: This formula refers to the method of fighting against weapons in the enemy's hands with my empty hands. When the enemy takes sharp weapons in his hands, no matter single or double, he must have one hand in the front and the other hand behind, so that he can only use one hand. Therefore, I only need to block his left hand and then his right hand will be useless. And when his right hand is blocked, his left hand will be useless. Generally, when only his front hand is blocked, his back hand will be useless. Even if his two hands come together, I only need to evade him, he will be completely useless, because he has no more hands.

18) Method of Pointing at the Mountain for Chipping Millstone

When his hand comes, my hand enters,
If I evade by angling the body, surely he will withdraw.
When he withdraws, my hand enters,
If he parries, my three attacks continue.

Annotation: The true aim of pointing at the mountain for chipping the millstone is towards the rock, not the mountain, because the rocks are the material for the millstone. Like the tactics of relieving the Zhao State by besieging the Wei State, the method of making a feint to the east while attacking in the west is applied. When this method is used, it is necessary to be calm in the mind and take the tactics of

Formulae

conquering the movement with stillness. If the enemy wants to punch me, I just turn the body to evade it and wait for a chance to attack back. Because he misses his strike, surely he will be eager to attack again quickly. When he moves his arm back, I can take advantage of his gesture to walk forward. Certainly, he will try to take the blocking method if he wants to evade me, then I can use the palm penetration to poke him continuously, giving him no time to breathe and he will be confused completely.

19) Method of Extricating Body for Becoming a Shadow

I call him in when he does not come,
I move away when he comes.
Not depending upon hands, just by body method,
Every step controlled by hips and waist.

Annotation: This formula talks about the unique characteristic of the Eight Diagram Palm and how to use the strategy of guerrilla warfare, which is that "when the enemy comes, I evade; when the enemy retreats, I pursue; when the enemy stops, I trouble him; when the enemy is fatigued, I attack him." In combat, if the power of both parties is equal and he also insists on the method of waiting for me to attack first, I must try my best to force him to play his hand. If he extends his hand, I just walk away. When he withdraws his hand, I just follow him and try to take the opportunity to attack him. You come and I go, not losing him and not fighting recklessly, but just playing with him. Usually, it depends upon the close coordination of the footwork and bodywork to find the opportunity, while the variation of the footwork and bodywork must be governed and accomplished by the waist and hips.

Liang Zhen Pu Eight Diagram Palm

20) Method of Turning Body to Flank

Extend the hand slightly and walk with big steps,
Open with half step for close-in capture.
Side step and lower the body to evade,
Capture when he wants to turn.

Annotation: In combat, Eight Diagram Palm always tries to move and turn behind the enemy to attack. This formula refers to the method of turning to flank the enemy. In attacking, the hand must extend with some force combined with a big step. However, in close quarters, smaller steps are required applying open steps with only a half step or shuffle and using striding steps to turn the opponent's corner. In this action it is necessary to lower the body in the turn. This is to avoid the enemy seizing as I move close to the side of his body. As he follows me in turning, I can apply the Eagle-Claw seizure tactics.

21) Method for Knocking, Pounding, Chopping and Bumping

When he strikes, I strike back first,
Change steps to stick with the left hand while pounding the right hand.
Pile the elbows as standing stake while chopping in,
The hands shake in circles while bumping in.

Annotation: While the opponent knocks in from the exterior, I can also knock him back. But I must strive to be the first. If the opponent pounds toward me, I can change the step to strike his hands with my left hand and then punch him with the gathered power. If the opponent tries to chop on my head, I can brace my elbows up as the standing stake and dissolve his force with the drilling power. If the hands become entangled in the opponent's play, regardless of one or both hands, I can put my hands above his and whip his hands in circles to decrease his power and at the same time try to take the chance to strike him with hip, shoulder, or elbow.

22) Half Circle Hand Method

Hand method in others is mostly in a straight line,
Walk a half step forward and wait leisurely.
Pointing straight forward for oblique punching,
It is still all right to walk another half step forward.

Annotation: When others attack me, they often come in a straight line. I need only to half step obliquely and the opponent will miss his strike. Even if the opponent points straight forward but punches obliquely, I can still use the previous method to walk a half step obliquely, so that he will miss his strike again. This is the Half Circle Hand Method. This footwork is the main method of avoiding a strong strike and spotting the weak point. By patiently following the enemy's gestures, I can detect my best opportunity to ensure victory.

23) Whole Circle Hand Method

I am in the center with enemies on four sides,
Going through the flowers to strike the willow either in the west or in the east.
No matter how the wind and cloud change in eight directions,
I remain still.

Liang Zhen Pu Eight Diagram Palm

Annotation: When I am under attack from all directions, I must be calm in the mind and behave like nothing is happening around me. If enemies are attacking from all sides, my gestures cannot be sluggish or empty but rather crisp and sudden so that I can confuse the enemies with a movement as difficult to track as a butterfly fluttering among the flowers. With the enemies puzzled and confused, I can deal with the front as well as the back. I can advance or retreat as I like. I can also evade the real attack when it comes and counter when opportunity presents itself. This is the best method to conquer the enemy by mixing the real and false according to individual situation and circumstance.

24) Heart-Eye Method

With the heart (mind) as a general and the eyes as weapons,
It is possible to conquer him with awareness.
It is highly prohibited to be dull in heart (mind) and careless in observation,
Leading to a great confusion of hands and feet.

Annotation: This formula refers to the abilities of the hand, eye, body and foot method and how they are closely coordinated. Whether training for health or battle, the hand, eyes, body, foot and method must be closely coordinated in disciplined concentration. Therefore, it is said that "the hand reaches while the eyes arrive, the eyes arrive with intention, the intention appears when *Qi* arrives and the power appears when *Qi* arrives." In accordance with the situation, the power must be released with vicious cruelty. Only cruel attacks and stable steps can conquer the enemy. Dull in the heart (mind) or careless in observation, can lead to confusion in the hands and feet and defeat can be expected.

Formulae

25) Staring Method

While knives and spears bustling in four directions,
As well as in dark night without moon.
Lower the body and stare around,
Surely to win if walking in crawling steps.

Annotation: This formula infers that when I am under attack from all directions, I must be brave and calm in the mind. And on a dark night without the moon, I must use an even lower stance and stare wide-eyed in order to observe the enemy in the dark of the night. For this the footwork must be lower to the ground to puzzle the enemy, then I can seek out the opportunity to attack with certainty.

26) Weapon Fighting Method

Although long, short, single and double weapons appear perfect,
They do not seem equal to two hands.
After iron palm is perfected as a weapon,
Bare hands can find the arm and wrist for fighting.

Annotation: Dealing with weapons with empty hands has been discussed in the seventeenth formula. Here I will discuss it further. Weapons occupy both hands and because I am empty handed, I am free and nimble. In skillful combat, the body must first avoid the attack by evading, jumping or moving; second, the palm method should be combined with a seizing method to "grasp and seal the blood vessels of the enemy and stop his motion." Specifically, we seek out the opponent's arm and wrist that wields the weapon and apply a palm strike, rendering his weapon useless. (Note: The meaning of the "iron palm" is descriptive. It means that the skill is highly refined. It does not literally mean skill achieved after practicing the "iron palm" method.)

27) Body Safeguarding Method

No need to boast about strong conquering weak,
It's a real skill if weak can conquer strong.
No matter how fast and hard an arrow leaves its bow,
Mistakes surely will not happen if rubbing the body.

Annotation: This formula is similar to the previous People Vanquishing Method and Half Circle Hand Method. It refers to the importance of strategic positioning. "Rubbing the body" refers to staying close to the body of the enemy, while flanking him, so that no matter how powerful or strong the enemy is, my body is out of direct danger.

28) Confusing the Enemy Method

To confuse his mind, first confuse his eyes,
Thousands of techniques are no better than one palm penetration.
Penetrate toward the nose continuously,
Alternate steps, moving left and right, to control the enemy.

Annotation: Puzzling the enemy begins when confusion is introduced to his eyes. Because the mind commands everything, in mental confusion it fails to direct the hands and feet. Therefore, it is necessary to puzzle the heart (mind) first, then without hesitation apply the penetrating palm with alternating steps, continuously toward the nose so that in his confusion he will be unable to deal with these strikes and victory will come quickly. "The best skills under heaven fear the three penetrations"; and "thousands of strokes are no better than a palm penetration," these two phrases refer directly to the terribleness of the stroke.

Formulae

29) Opening Closing Method

It is common to open first in hope of closing,
When seeing his opening, prevent closing.
A comeback will be staged in pretense of failure,
Meanings are implied in pointing to the east while striking west.

Annotation: This formula emphasizes the importance of mastering the strategies and tactics of combat. All boxing skills include opening and closing. Generally, the enemy creates an opening just prior to his closing in attack. Therefore, in combat, as soon as the opponent's opening is spotted, we should move quickly to prevent his closing. If the opponent's force has not been completely expended in this attempt, we must induce him to attack again. This can be accomplished by a pretense of vulnerability. This is the principle of pointing to the east but attacking the west to create an opening.

30) South Orientating Method

No matter how swift his thousands of hand and eyes are,
It's natural to safeguard the center.
Don't extend the hand if not necessary,
The hand should be able to return after it is extended.

Annotation: Even when the opponent is attacking in countless strikes and from various angles, I only have to protect the center. In dealing with the numerous strikes, my hands should stay close to my body to provide constant protection and not extend away from my body unless absolutely necessary and even then should be retracted as soon as possible. In combat, it is preferable to survey the area for obstacles and pitfalls and to seek the flat ground and favorable terrain for stance and maneuvers. One should also take notice of atmospheric conditions. Don't stand with the sun shining in your face. Wind and wetness should also be considered.

31) Approaching Method

Blocking is a body safeguarding skill,
Evading others with casual poise.
When distance is more than half Chi (1/3 meter) away,
Skills will be useless and effort wasted.

Annotation: "Neither too close nor too far" is a boxing axiom that reflects the point of this formula. Supreme skill would allow me to block in a manner appearing casual and effortless. This is described as "bravery founded in skillfulness." But it is necessary to be close to the enemy's body to execute the blocks, no more than 1/3 meter. If too far away, the venture to secure advantageous leverage and control would be as futile as lighting a lamp for a blind man.

32) Six Direction Method

Six Direction Method in others is empty talk,
My palm method reflects the principle of six directions.
Moving one step will attend to eight directions,
It is not difficult to look forward and pay attention to the back at the same time.

Annotation: The arts of attacking skills emphasize how to observe the six directions and monitor the eight directions. The six directions refer to the front, back, left, right, upper and lower directions. The eight directions refer to the four cardinal directions of the east, south, west and north and four diagonal directions of the southeast, southwest, northeast and northwest. The footwork of circle walking in the Eight-Diagram Palm makes it easy to observe and monitor the eight directions. One glance while stepping enables one to see the whole circle. Therefore, it is naturally easy to look forward and monitor behind at the same time.

Formulae

33) Only Way Method

Don't punch rashly if not accurate,
Punch again if one is misses.
Even if he is as nimble as a ghost or god,
Don't let it shake your spirit.

Annotation: The arts of attack emphasize "stable, accurate and cruel." Therefore, it is necessary to be accurate in striking. If uncertain, better to withhold the striking, i.e. don't shoot the arrow without a target, because you will be leaving yourself open for no true advantage. But, however, if you should strike and, by chance, miss, you should continue to strike again and again in close order so that you leave no time for the opponent to evade and set himself up to counter. Sometimes when you shoot again and again, constant as the waves on the shore, the opponent will panic rendering his skillful hands and feet useless.

34) Slip Preventing Method

It is difficult to hold steps in ice and snow-covered ground,
Stepping forward, backward, side or straight, the heart is quiet.
Small steps are required for rotation,
Avoid stiffening the body and striking high.

Annotation: The sum and substance is in the last sentence: "Avoid stiffening the body and striking high." Because the center of balance goes upward in the upper body, the lower part can easily slip out from underneath, which, generally, invites disaster by tumbling and, therefore, is highly prohibited.

Liang Zhen Pu Eight Diagram Palm

35) Step Stabilizing Method

The body will sway if the steps are unstable,
That toes can grasp solid ground will be better than thousands of strokes.
Walk forward with the toes and backward by lifting the heel,
Don't turn around without kou step.

Annotation: This is a continuation of the previous song. This formula discusses various aspects of the footwork. The first sentence indicates the danger in unstable footwork, that is, the tendency for the whole body to be unstable if the foot is unstable. The second sentence indicates the benefits in the stable step, referring to the forceful effect of the whole body power in applying strokes which requires the toes and feet to grasp solid ground. This whole body power is what renders the technique "better than thousands of strokes." The third sentence comments on the method for advance and retreat, that is, that the toes must grasp the ground in advancing the steps and hook the step (*kou bu*) before turning and walking in the opposite direction. This refers to the so-called "toe-in" or "T-stance". It warns not to begin to turn without this kou step first in place. This is a key to stability and swift turning.

36) Ten Step Method

Walk small steps when turning the body,
With big steps the body is not coordinated and the footwork is not agile.
Turning the body in half steps,
It is difficult for others to catch me and know my intention.

Annotation: The foot method, a vital component in the boxing skills, requires the nimble and active movement and turning in both advancing and retreating. The small stepping method is necessary for

Formulae

the nimble and active qualities. Large steps combined with fast movements would cause clumsy movement in turning. Not only are you not in fine control of yourself, but at the same time it is easy to be sensed by the opponent. In combat, the steps should be appropriately shortened so that it is easy to approach the enemy and difficult for him to sense my intention and resist the attacks.

37) Palm Method

Although palm skill is divided into upper, middle and lower,
The upper and lower parts are just a frame.
Only the middle part can guarantee free rotation,
From which changes in upper and lower parts take place.

Annotation: All kinds of the boxing methods talk about the skills in the upper, middle and lower parts, which respectively refer to the high gesture, middle gesture and lower gestures. The high gestures conserve energy, while lower gestures require more energy. In training, it is necessary to work the lower gestures as much as possible, for attaining skills. In combat, however, it is proper to hold the middle position, which enables the body to rotate smoothly and freely, so that all the changes are coordinated from the middle position. Because all the changes in the upper and middle parts are obtained from the smooth and free rotation of the waist and hips, it is said that it is the middle part "from which changes in upper and lower parts take place."

38) Forward Bending Prohibiting Method

To bow the head equals closing the eyes,
The body would fall forward as well.
Lowering the head and bending the waist causes death of the middle axis,
So that whole foot and whole palm cannot be used.

Annotation: All kinds of boxing skills prohibit bowing the head and bending the waist both in training or in combat. When the head bends, it is not possible to see in front. This is the same as closing the eyes. When the body bends, the middle axis is bent, and it is not possible to turn and twist freely. Also due to the forward leaning posture, it is easy for the body to fall forward. In such a situation, how are you able to deal with the enemy? Therefore, it is said in the boxing proverbs that bending the head and waist creates problems in the eight gestures. Although the boxing methods of the hand, eyes, body and feet are discussed and theorized, it is not enough to work out all the mysteries in attacking arts. Only by combining the mind, Qi and power, and practicing both the internal and external is it possible to realize true skill. If the head is bowed and the waist is bent, it is impossible to have a smooth mind and Qi, hindering all the strokes attempted. Without complete control of the four limbs, which is directed by the waist, hand and foot methods would be useless. Therefore, the waist and the head must be free for turning and when the knee is flexed, the kneecap cannot go past the foot and the head cannot go past the knees.

39) Backward Moving Prohibiting Method

Silent stillness is sought in spread back and hollow chest,
To not correctly hold the chest and belly brings regret.
It is not possible to hold the waist inward when the belly is thrown out,
Terrible fear is created when the body cannot rotate freely.

Annotation: The Eight Diagram Palm is an internal boxing skill that seeks movement from stillness. Therefore, during training and combat, it is required to spread the back and hollow the chest for Qi to descend into the Dantian area. When Qi is smooth, the mind can be calm. This is why the first sentence in Master Dong Hai Chuan's songs says to "empty the chest, erect the neck and lower the waist." Because the calm mind can help to observe the enemy clearly, it becomes possible to take the proper method to deal with the enemy. If the chest and belly are thrust outward and the body gravity is inclined, it is easy to fall

Formulae

backward. Although the benefits in holding the waist inward are understood, it is not possible to use them if the chest and belly are thrust out (forward). In particular, the restricted rotation and movement would interfere with applying the body method.

40) Vertical Body Method

The power of whole body lies in the middle axis,
The power is different with body in slant.
No matter how you bend the legs, the body remains straight,
Extend the hand like an arrow without stopping.

Annotation: A primary rule in internal boxing is to keep the body stable and centered. Because the power of the whole body is in the waist, regardless of the movement, rotation and power release, everything is in the waist and hips. Therefore, it is said "controlled and governed by the waist." Consequently, the body must stay centered, without leaning forward or backward. Although the steps are moving, the body should always be kept vertical. Even when the power is released in combat, the body should be kept vertical to move forward. If the body leans, the ability to release power will be greatly reduced. Therefore, in order to have a powerful release, the lower part must be stable and the body vertical.

41) Body Supplementing Method

The body is like a king and the waist and legs are ministers,
An upright king and strong ministers can conquer enemies.
Advance, retreat and evasion all depend upon body method,
No spirit will be produced without the waist and legs.

Annotation: In the Vertical Body Method, it is required to maintain a centered vertical body alignment, which allows for active and free movement and turning that easily combines the waist and legs for producing power for combat. All the methods of advance, retreat and evasion in the boxing skills are coordinated by the body method. But the accomplishment of the body method relies upon the coordination of the four limbs, especially the coordination of the waist and legs. Therefore, it is said that "there is no polishing of skills without the waist and legs."

42) Body Turning Method

If the opponent approaches to conquer me,
When my hands and feet cannot prevail.
I turn the body to either side accordingly,
To turn danger into safety and capture him.

Annotation: The Body Turning Method is the unique law of the Eight-Diagram Palm. At the moment when the enemy attacks me, punches to my chest with the right fist, if it is too late for me to use my handwork and footwork, I can hollow my chest and turn the waist to the right, so that it is possible to flank the enemy on the right. If he punches me with the left fist, I can turn left to his left flank. In this way, I am able to turn danger into safety and to seize an opportunity to conquer him.

43) Step Walking and Body Turning Method

A forceful direct attack is difficult to stop,
The first attack has the advantage.
Retreating continuously in a fight against an opponent,
Is not as good as side stepping and turning the body.

Formulae

Annotation: A lively attack in combat often cannot be resisted. If I am unable to deal with the attack, it is advisable to evade. But if the opponent continues to attack, one can merely side step and turn the body, so that the opponent will miss his strike. This formula is similar to the Half Circle Hand Method.

44) Body Swinging Method

Come west after evading east,
Shake the body and make a change.
Do the same on both sides,
Pushing forward and pulling backward are coordinated by
the waist.

Annotation: There are two meanings in this formula. First, when I am alone facing a group of the enemies, it is surely difficult to deal with them when they come in the west again after I evade them in the east. At that moment, it is advisable to take the active method of "going through the flowers and striking the willow," and penetrate the attackers forward then strike them backward. Second, if alone and the opponent is fast in hands and powerful in force in attacking me, I just turn my body, walk behind him and attack him, strike him and throw him with whole body power.

45) Step Squatting and Body Lowering Method

It's surely difficult to raise the hands and parry blows,
In the upper part with tall and big opponents.
It is necessary to bend legs and lower body,
Inducing him into my trap where methods can be used freely.

Liang Zhen Pu Eight Diagram Palm

Annotation: In combat with a tall, big man, certainly I would suffer a lot if I played with him in the high postures. Therefore, I need to induce him to use the lower gestures. When I squat my body down, surely he will follow me and squat down. I am then free to use high, middle and low positions while he is only left with the middle and low positions. Consequently, my disadvantage becomes my advantage. Hence, the phrase "inducing him into my trap where methods can be used freely."

46) Capture Prohibiting Method

Eight diagram hand does not talk of grabbing,
My skill is not superior if I grab a person.
With multiple opponents it is not appropriate,
Best to employ direct attack and direct withdraw.

Annotation: The Eight Diagram Palm does not advocate to conquer the opponent by the capture method. Since the capture method can only deal with one person at a time, and then my two hands are occupied and not free to use against others, it is not a superior skill in dire circumstances. Therefore, it is said that "my skill is not superior if I grab a person." Facing a group of enemies alone this method would prove ineffective and it would be much better to deal with a group of them through direct attack and immediate withdraw.

47) Stand Prohibiting Method

Walk without limitation for mixing all into one force,
Implies the eight diagram principle of my family.
Every technique depends upon changes in steps,
Still standing is like a flower on the ground.

Formulae

Annotation: The skills in the Eight Diagram Palm are obtained by walking and the principles of the Eight Diagram Palm are constant movement and change and cultivation of *Qi*. Therefore, walking and turning must be combined with the Taoist breathing techniques. Hence, it is possible to consolidate all the forces into one. This is achieved by persistent walking. Therefore, it is said that "walking is the foundation of all the skills, no skills are better than walking." The way to deal with the enemy in the Eight Diagram Palm depends upon the circle walking, puzzling the enemy and defeating them by circle walking. If you stand still, it is easy to be defeated, like a flower on the ground is easily trampled. Consequently, the stationery stance is highly prohibited, and the practitioners must understand the importance of the constant walking.

48) Ultimate Method

Power must be full and techniques must be accurate,
No mess of three even if a blow is missed.
There is no limit in strokes within strokes,
Spiritual method can be sought in pure hands.

Annotation: The highest stage of the methods and skills are described as the supreme and absolute skills. The formula implies that the Eight Diagram Palm is the most refined art in the boxing skills. There are more specific methods and skills which are not found in other boxing arts. Therefore, it is referred to as the Ultimate Method. Although the methods and skills in the Eight Diagram Palm are supreme, it is still necessary to cultivate the proper power, which is precisely the whole body power previously described. Also, it is necessary to be calm in the mind and brave in spirit for striking accurately. But, what can we do if the target is missed and the power is lost due to the mistakes in the estimation? Still we should be calm, so that the mind, hands and feet will not be in a mess. This is the so-called "no mess of the three." Further, we can observe the enemy and change our gestures according to his variations. It is possible to strike in accordance with the principle of the movement and change in the eight diagrams, so that the continuous strikes make it difficult for the opponent to deal with us. But, this state of the unpredictable changes can only be obtained by the close and correct coordination of the hands, eyes, body and methods, combined with the internal essence, *Qi* and spirit, and pure and proficient skills. At that moment, nothing is unattainable.

Formula Verse

Real meanings are implied in forty-eight methods,
Spirit will not appear just by speaking and practicing,
If real and pure skills are expected to be obtained,
Three years experiment must be undertaken among several people.

Annotation: The forty-eight songs are the training methods of the Eight Diagram Palm and the rules that must be followed have profound results. It takes at least three years of correct practice to properly understand the essentials of the Eight Diagram Palm for obtaining the integrated internal and external skills. The methods for the practice generally can be described in four points. The first point is the observation. First, one should observe how the teacher practices and then imitate the gestures. Afterwards, one should observe how others practice and consider whether their methods are appropriate or not for improving one's own skills. Then, one should study others writings for a better understanding of the theory. The second point is listening. First listen to the teacher's instruction and then to the experiential insights of schoolmates to improve one's own practice. The third point is thinking. Thinking over the best way to discard the crude and to retain the essential for improvement. The fourth point is practice. Persistent practice is a necessary component, because the practice of internal boxing skills is a painstaking and complicated work. The real skills can only be obtained through the extensive practice. Because there is no shortcut, the practice cannot be rash and must be carefully studied. Therefore, it requires a long-term plan for developing the internal boxing skills. An old proverb says: "It is easy to practice the boxing skill, but difficult to understand its theory." Another says: "One thousand practices make the theory understood." Therefore, it is necessary to first develop proper boxing skills and all the experiences that it entails in order to develop the hindsight required for complete understanding of the theory. "If real and pure skills are expected to be obtained, a three year effort must be undertaken among several people." This refers to the necessity of first a proper teacher, then training partners and, finally, other opinions.

    The forty-eight methods are the applied methods of the Eight Diagram Palm. The teacher puts in proper place the skills of the hand, eye, body method and footwork as well as the internal essence, Qi and spirit. However, if how to deal with an enemy is not studied, it is still possible to be in a great bustle of the hands and feet and unable to deal with the enemy in practical application. Therefore, it is necessary to play with others often for obtaining the practical experience. The practical experience of battle is much more difficult than ordinary practice. It may take seven or eight years of continuous effort to accumulate sufficient experience to apply the methods. Because only by perfect proficiency, can the skills be used freely at anytime so that you can do whatever you want with your skills, and defeat any kind of enemy.

Endnotes

    [1]The specific repositioning of the foot's angle of articulation at the ankle as well as from the hip and knee.

    [2]Spirit could mean energy level and does mean energy level, which could be more in reference to basic vitality level. Or it could mean mental alertness and intensity which could be more in reference to a combative environment.

    [3]This stamp is not necessarily a highly visible percussive action with audible sound effects but rather a sudden downward thrusting of the root that can be invisibly sublime and inaudible as well.

Liang Zhen Pu Eight Diagram Palm

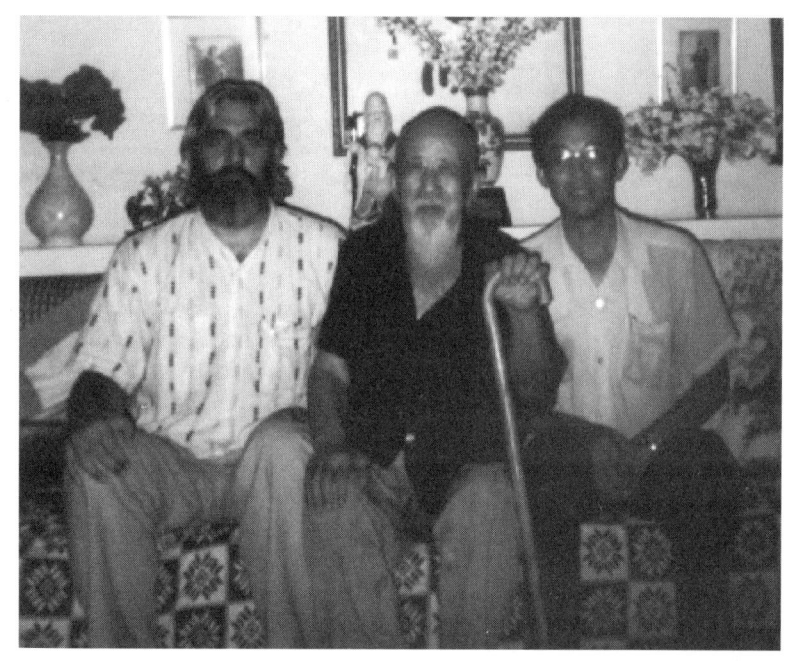

Li Tzu Ming with his students Vince Black and Zhao Da Yuan

CHAPTER VI

EXERCISES AND FIGURES OF EIGHT DIAGRAM PALM

The Eight Diagram Palm introduced in this chapter, one of the oldest eight diagram palm methods, is usually referred to as the "Old Eight Palms." During compilation, we have tried out best to provide the precise descriptions and illustrations. Concerning the figures, a minimum of figures of the movements and gestures are included in order to avoid obstructing the movement lines and preserve their continuity. The lines drawn in the figures of the hands and feet designate the next movement of the hands and feet. The order of the foot movements are indicated by the numbers.

As for the visual angle in the figure drawing, the angle of the steps in the figures may be slightly different in actual practice and there may be some deviation in the direction. Therefore, the literal explanation is presented forthwith. (Note: The photographs of Mr. Zhao Da Yuan, one of Li Zi Ming's top students, which appear in this chapter did not appear in the original book. This new addition to the English translation was added for clarity.)

The Old Eight Palms, also called the Eight Mother Palms, are the basic palm skills of Eight Diagram Palm, in which the Single Palm Change is the fundamental gesture. The circle walking gesture in the Single Palm Change, traditionally called the "millstone pushing" gesture, occupies a very special position in Eight Diagram Palm. It is absolutely necessary for beginners to master the exercises of the millstone pushing gesture. It is explained in the following:

Training Area

Initially, select a level area approximately 2.5 meters in diameter. Beginners are instructed to inscribe a circle on the ground and then walk along the border of the circle for the turning and changing of the postures.

Liang Zhen Pu Eight Diagram Palm

Opening Gesture of Eight-Diagram Palm

Preparatory stance:

Stand on northern border of the circle and face the center of the circle (due south) with the heel together and toes separated to an angle of approximately 60°. The knees are together, hips are held under tilting the tailbone slightly. The back is straight and vertical and the chest is hollowed. The shoulders are relaxed and drooping down toward the ribs with the arms hanging the hands naturally at the thighs while the neck is held upright but without tension of any kind. The head is held up from the vertex as though suspended on a string and the lower jaw is drawn slightly inward. The mouth is naturally closed with the tongue curled to touch the roof of the mouth and all breathing is performed through the nose. Calm the mind and maintain deep natural breathing.

Explanation of millstone pushing gesture (left gesture):

1) Turn to the right (45° to 60°), the foot angles open about 30° each from the circle arc. The upper body maintains unmoved.

2) Lower the body, bend the knees keeping them close together, shift the weight to the right leg, and lift the left leg slightly. As the body squats down, turn the waist to the right side as far as possible, rotate the right palm outward (ending with the palm facing up) and push it forward and up to the level of the chin, at the same time rotating the left palm outward (to palm up position) and thrusting it toward the right ribs along the waist and abdomen. As the eyes turn to look left, move the left side forward on the perimeter of the circle by extending the left foot forward while thrusting the left penetrating palm forward from under the right elbow up to the height of the nose. At the last instant of extending the palm the left foot should find its root.

3) Continuing from the above movement, as the eyes look to the left, turn the waist to the left simultaneously, the left palm (with the palm upward and extending up and forward) swinging to the left with the waist rotation. The right palm also follows the left-turning waist to the left. When the palms are pointing to the center of the circle, the two palms turn inward simultaneously, the left palm drops at the wrist with the palm turning toward the center of the circle (the thumb is curved, creating a crescent shape between the thumb and index finger, the other

Exercises and Figures

fingers are straight and slightly spread to form a hollow in the palm), the palm remains vertical and thumb and index finger are held at the level of the eyebrows. While the right palm is turning inward, simultaneously drop the shoulder, elbow and wrist to the lower border of the left ribs (the right palm obliquely faces the center of the circle), while the two arms retain their rounded form. In general, when turning to the left the legs stay flexed or bent and the body weight remains slightly inclined on the right leg, maintain a constant height when turning the body left as much as possible and keep the back round and the right palm coordinated directly above the right heel. The eyes stare at the tips of the middle and index fingers of the left palm. This posture is traditionally called the left millstone pushing gesture of the middle part. See Figure 1-1.

As far as internal images, one should mentally embrace the chicken leg, dragon body, monkey shape, bear shoulder, tiger crouch and leopard head. These images serve to imbue their qualities into the physical movements and postures.

Section 1 - Single Palm Change

Movement explanation:

1) The Single Palm Change starts from the left millstone pushing gesture while walking counter clockwise as shown in Figure 1-1.

2) To implement the Single Palm Change the outside foot (right foot while moving counter clockwise) steps forward on the circle in a toe-in position resulting in an inward splay-foot stance with the two knees close together. After placing the right foot, immediately turn the body to the left rotating the left arm externally (with the palm up) and simultaneously rotate the right arm outward so the palm is up. The eyes stare at the left hand. See Figure 1-2.

3) The right foot steps straight ahead on the circle so that the body in effect has turned to face the left side and the stance is in a outward or complex splay-foot. As the right foot is stepping forward on the circle, the right palm simultaneous penetrates forward from beneath the left elbow and forearm with the palm and fingers pointing forward and the thumb curved slightly. (The penetrating palm keeps all the fingers close together piling up against each other with the palm slightly cupped and the thumb locked in on the palmar base of the index finger.) This leaves Hukou upward in a standing palm hand position. The left palm also turns inward at the same time, the wrist turning down resulting in a

Liang Zhen Pu Eight Diagram Palm

standing palm below the right elbow. At this moment, the face and chest are facing the opposite direction of the original left millstone pushing gesture. See Figure 1-3.

4) Then the right palm follows the right turning waist to move upward to the right then curving slightly downward to drop on the right side (the palm facing the center of the circle, with the shoulder, elbow and wrist sunken downward and the finger tip at the level of the eyebrow). The left palm also follows the waist turning slightly inward to stop near the medial side of the right elbow (the palm faces to the center of the circle obliquely), the eyes look at the right palm to form the right millstone pushing gesture, as shown in Figure 1-4.

In other words, after the right palm penetration, turn the body to the right to form the right millstone pushing gesture. This sequence remains the same through out the exercise.

The above explanation is the exercise to turn the left millstone-pushing gesture into the right millstone pushing gesture (single palm change). The Eight-Diagram Palm gestures to the right as well as the left. The right gesture should be practiced after the left gesture. In order to decrease the length of this presentation and avoid repetition, all the movement explanations will introduce the left rotating gestures and how they are performed, while the right-rotating gesture and exercises are omitted. All movements are bilateral, the right handed gestures are being omitted for the sake of clarity in presentation and can be worked out by the practitioners themselves. The following gestures are the same.

Main Points

1) All the movements should be in coordination and embracing the six harmonies, i.e. chicken leg, dragon body, etc.

2) When turning to one side the lead arm should extend forward and the crossing rear arm should root its power in the shoulder, sinking the shoulder and elbow and curving the arm so that it is neither extended completely straight or bent too much and *Hukou* is still rounded.

3) Slightly embrace the two thighs, embrace the arms, lift the anus, keep the knees close and curve the legs, hollowing the chest while maintaining a vertical spine and the *Qi* sinks into Dantian while the eyes remain alert.

4) The hooking steps (*kou bu*) must be distinctive and the foot must not scrape the ground in stepping.

Exercises and Figures

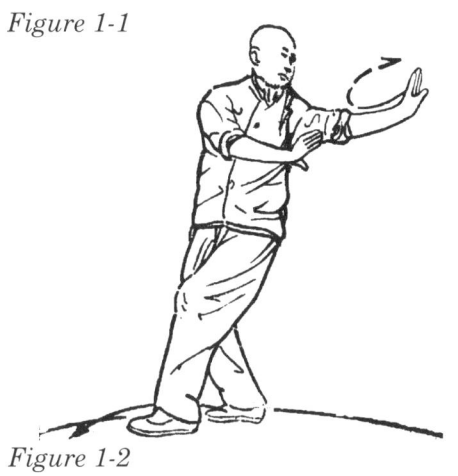

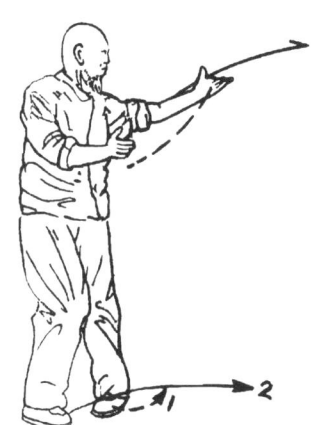

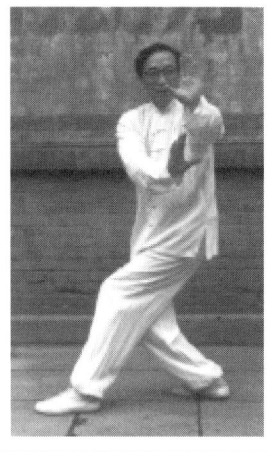

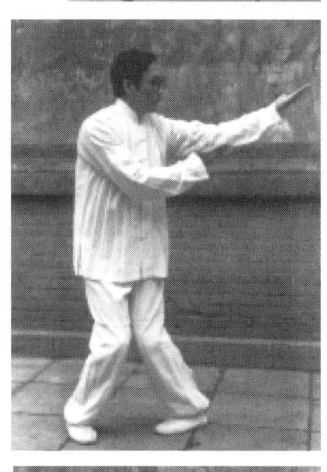

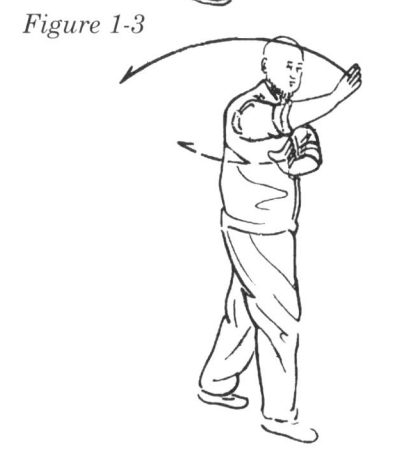

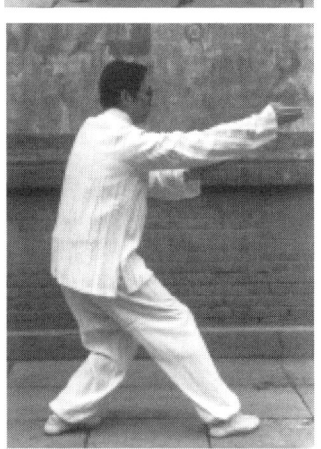

Figure 1-1

Figure 1-2

Figure 1-3

115

Liang Zhen Pu Eight Diagram Palm

Figure 1-4

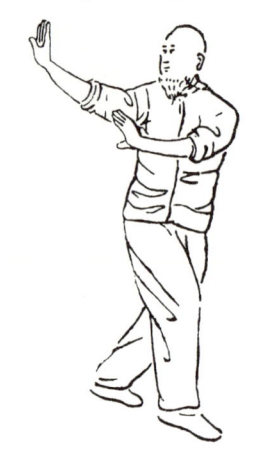

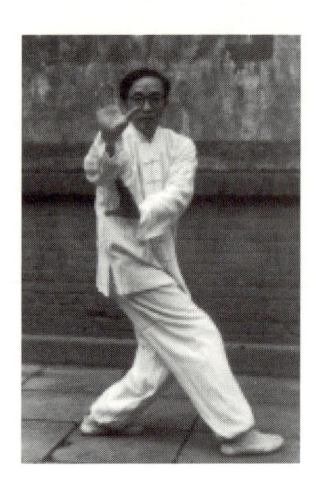

Section 2 - Double Palm Change

Movement Explanation

1) Double Palm Change is also termed the Covering Palm. It starts to turn to the left from the left millstone pushing gesture of the Single Palm Change, as shown in Figure 2-1.

2) Starting from the same position as the beginning of the form, that is, the first left millstone pushing gesture. The right foot walks a step forward on the circle, the right and the upper body remain unmoved and the body gravity moves to the right leg. Then the left foot kicks forward to the right side (not higher than the waist, with the dorsum of the foot stretched flat). The left palm drops in front of the left side when the left foot begins to kick, following the dropping gesture, the left palm moves down and back and over the top to the front in a circle, and then the left palm slaps the dorsum of the left foot exactly when the left foot kicks upward, as shown in Figure 2-2.

3) Continuing, the left foot kicks backward and drops behind the right foot and the two feet form a reversed splay-foot. At the same time, the left palm also follows, when the left foot drops, moving downward to the left with the ulnar side of the palm up. The eyes watch over the left shoulder, the right palm and the left palm spread at the same time with the thumbs of the two hands downward. The chest faces toward the circle, as shown in Figure 2-3.

4) In conjunction with the above movements, the right foot first hooks inward and the left foot turns outward, the weight shifts to the left foot, and the right foot steps forward. While stepping forward, the left palm turns inward lightly to have the palm center down, and then the left palm continues to move forward and to the centerline. At the same time, the right palm supinates while moving to the front of the chest then penetrate beneath the left forearm. When the right penetrating palm crosses underneath the left elbow, the left arm will draw into its root and the shoulder will sink and pull the left arm suddenly in a backward motion while the right shoulder projects the right penetrating palm suddenly forward. See figure 2-4.

5) Following the previous gesture, the right foot hooks inward (the inward rotation and the body turns to the left (facing outside the circle), then the left foot swings into external rotation and simultaneously the right palm rotates outward to have the palm center upward. Then the right foot walks one step forward into a right bow step, at the same time, the right palm following the movement rotates in pronation arcing over the head to press down in front. At this moment, the right palm center moves obliquely downward, the left palm center faces downward, the left palm is on the right axillary side with the eyes watching the right hand, as shown in Figure 2-5.

6) Following the previous movement, while the body turns to the left the left foot swings rotating outward and stands firmly on the circle, at the same time, the left palm supinates up and out to the left anterior in a standing palm (the finger tips toward the left front), the right palm moves to the right waist, as shown in Figure 2-6.

7) The right foot steps straight ahead on the circle so that the body in effect has turned to face the left side and the stance is in a outward or complex splay-foot. As the right foot is stepping forward on the circle, the right palm simultaneously penetrates forward from beneath the left elbow and forearm with the palm and fingers pointing forward and the thumb curved slightly. This leaves Hukou upward in a standing palm position. The left palm also turns inward at the same time. The wrist turning down results in a standing palm below the right elbow. At this moment the face and chest are facing the opposite direction of the original left millstone pushing gesture. See Figure 2-7.

8) Then the right palm follows the right turning waist to move upward to the right and curves slightly downward to drop on the right side (the palm facing the center of the circle, with the shoulder, elbow and wrist sunken downward and the finger tip at the level of the eyebrow). The left palm also follows the waist turning slightly inward and to stop near the medial side of the right elbow (the palm faces to the center of the

Liang Zhen Pu Eight Diagram Palm

circle obliquely), the eyes look at the right palm to form the right millstone pushing gesture.

Main Points

   1) In kicking the left foot, the point of force is either the foot tip or the dorsum of the foot. The leg is slightly flexed and the foot tip shouldn't be too high and usually is at the level of the waist.

   2) On slapping the palm, the two arms extend outward to the both sides, but the arms should be curved round and not extended straight. The point of force of the two hands are on the ulnar edge of the palm.

   3) All the movements should be coordinated. Please refer to the first palm for other related information.

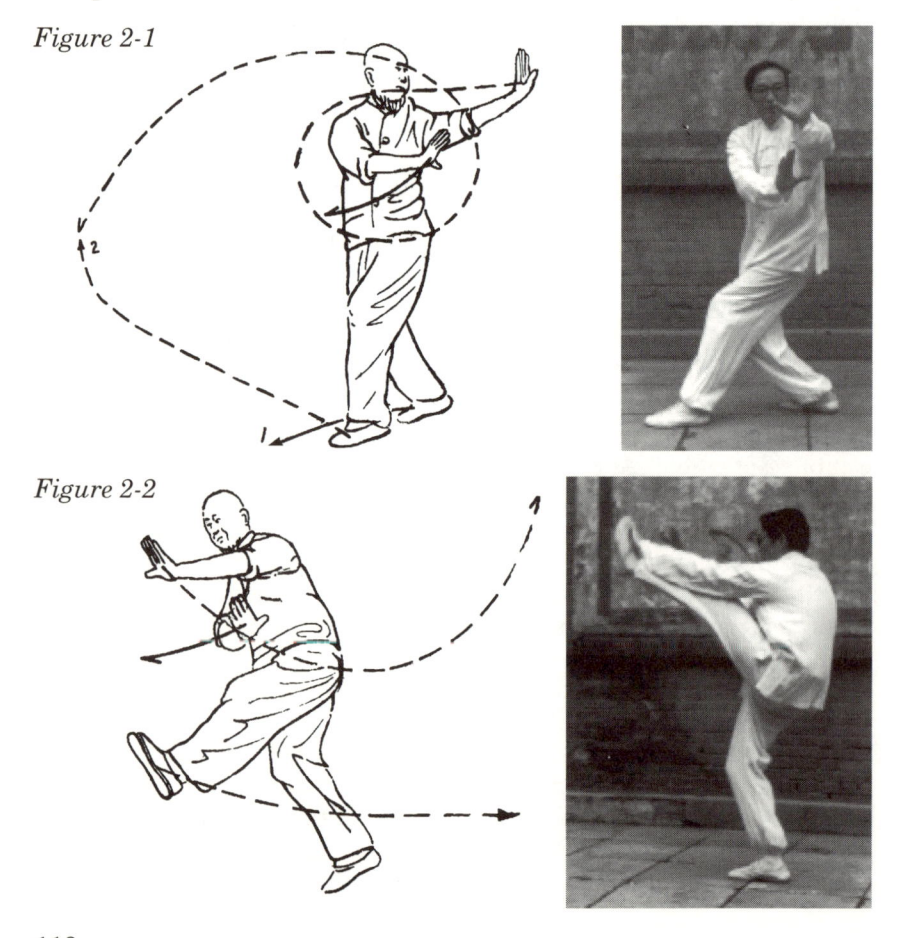

Figure 2-1

Figure 2-2

Exercises and Figures

Figure 2-3

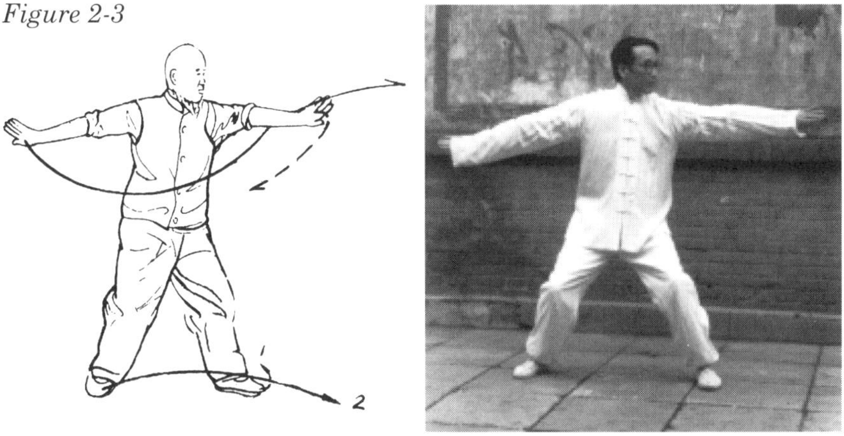

Figure 2-4

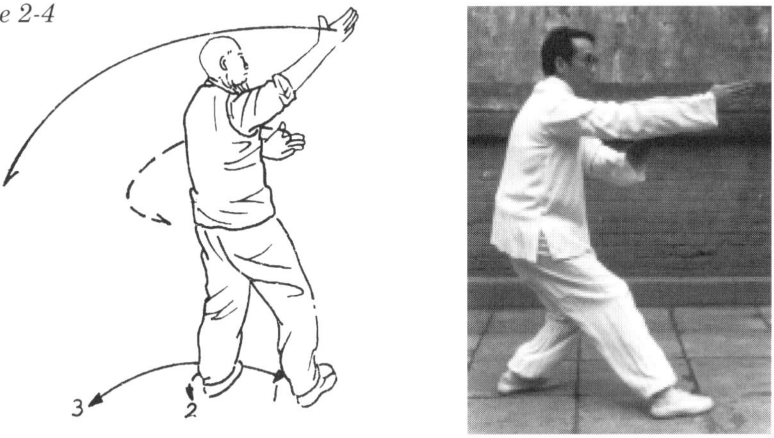

Figure 2-5

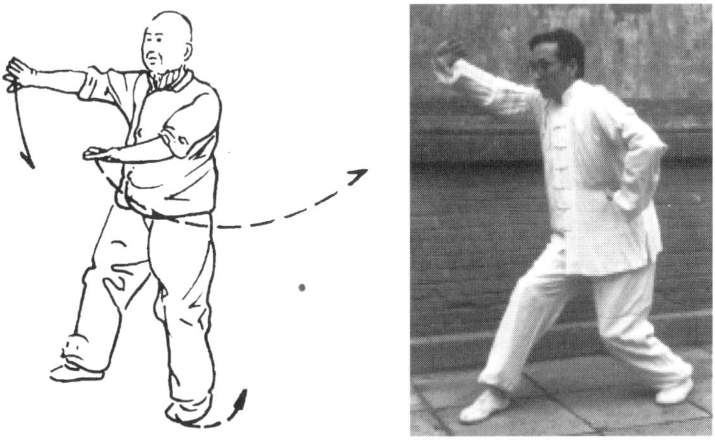

119

Liang Zhen Pu Eight Diagram Palm

Figure 2-6

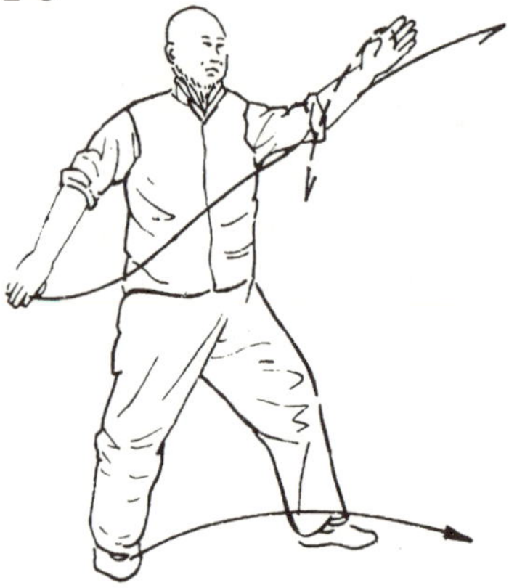

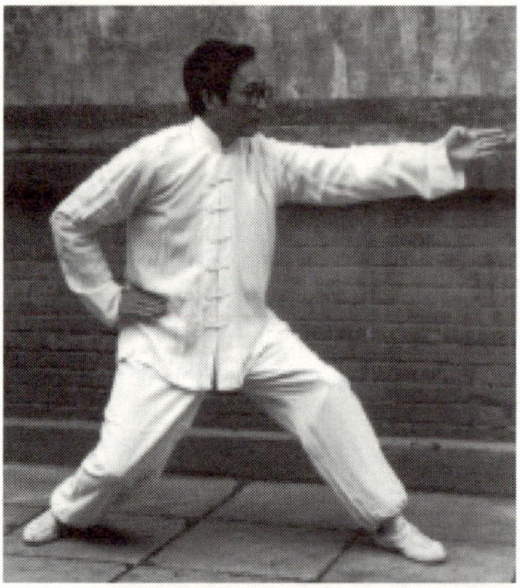

Figure 2-7

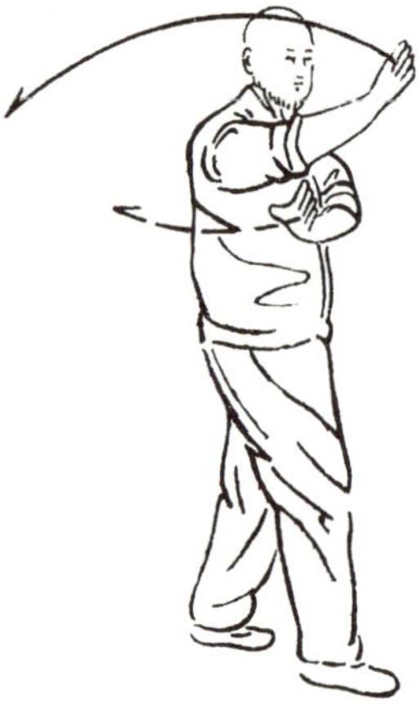

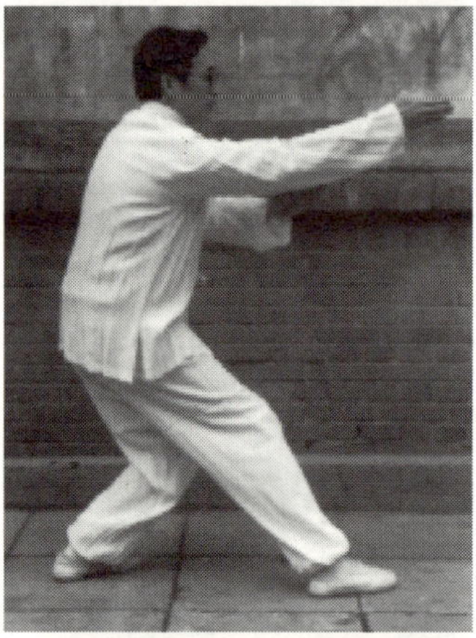

Figure 2-8

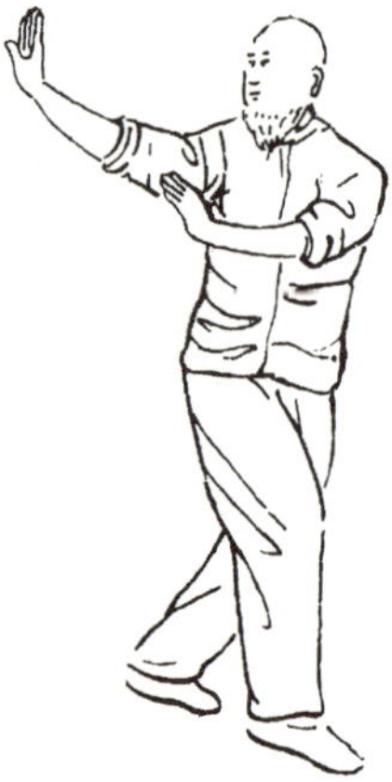

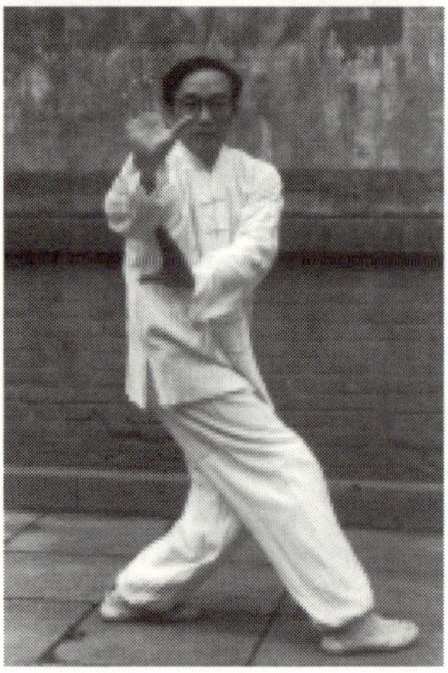

120

Exercises and Figures

Section 3 - Body Rotating Palm

Movement Explanation

1) The Body Rotating Palm, also called the Back Turning Palm, begins in the left millstone pushing gesture, as shown in Figure 3-1.

2) The waist turns the upper body to the right without altering the upper gesture. In this movement the right foot steps forward and splays the step outward as much as possible in complex splay-foot form. The body turns to the right and the left palm thrusts across the chest while the right palm thrusts underneath the left armpit with the palm downward. The left palm continues to follow the turning body (in a clockwise direction) and spirals around to set above the right elbow (with the palm downward), the eyes follow the left hand, the two knees gather together and the body moves downward slightly, as shown in Figure 3-2.

3) Then the left foot moves from in front of the right foot to behind the right foot (to the previous placement of the right foot hooking inward as much as possible), the body follows the step in turning 360° (facing the northwest), at the same time the two palms move from the front of the chest up, back, down and forward in dual arcs (of 2/3 meter in diameter) on both the left and the right and setting in front of the lower abdomen. The two palms touch each other at the base of the palms, with the thumbs and palm center forward and forming a forked double palm gesture. At this point, the palms rotate outward and the right foot tip is straight on the circle line and the right foot lunges forward with the left foot following and simultaneously the two palms push out forward, the weight on the left leg with the chest hollowed, sinking shoulders and elbows and contract the arms, as shown in Figure 3-3 (the interim movement) and Figure 3-4.

4) Then, the left foot moves around the front of the right foot and back behind the right foot, hooks inward as much as possible, and forms a complex splay-foot. The right foot turns outward to form a reverse splayfoot stance, then the body turns 270° to the right (facing the circle). While turning the body right, the form in the palms do not change and the two palms push upward (in front of the lower jaw, in a White Ape Pushing Gesture, with the palm center upward and the thumbs inward), with the body slightly sunken and the eyes watching both palms, as shown in Figure 3-5.

Liang Zhen Pu Eight Diagram Palm

5) Then, the left foot circles around the front and back to the rear of the right foot and hooks the step inward as much as possible, forming a complex splay-foot. Then the body turns clockwise with a left step in 360° (facing the circle), and afterwards the right foot steps to the right into a horse stance. At the same time, the two palms respectively press and strike first the left then the right (the palm center obliquely downward), as shown in Figure 3-6.

6) Then the right foot retreats one step to the right rear, the left foot follows the right foot to move one step forward, the left foot floating in an anterior false step with the body squatting low (facing the circle) and the weight on the right leg. At the same time, the right palm moves slightly downward, the left palm rotates outward and curves forward and then the hand moves out in front of the chest (with the palm upward), so that the left hand is in front of the left foot. The eyes watch the left hand, as shown in Figure 3-7.

7) Then, the left hand continues to rotate inward and downward to the side of the left hip (with the palm downward). At the same time, the left foot retreats one step to the left rear, the right foot follows the gesture to move one step to the front of the left foot, floating in a right anterior false step, and with the body squatting low (facing the circle) and the body gravity on the left leg. At the same time, the left palm moves in slightly downward and the right palm rotates outward and curves forward and then the hand moves out in front of the chest (with the palm upward). The right hand is in front of the right foot and the eyes watch the right hand, as shown in Figure 3-8.

8) Then, the right hand continues to rotate inward and downward to the side of the right hip (with the palm downward). At the same time, the right foot retreats one step to the right rear and the left foot follows the gesture to move one step to the front of the right foot, floating and with the body squatting low and the weight on the left leg. At the same time, the right palm moves in slightly downward and the left palm rotates outward and curves forward and then the hand moves out in front of the chest (with the palm upward), as shown in Figure 3-9.

9) Then, the left foot advances one step to the left along the circle line. The right palm does not move and the left palm rotates inward and downward, and slaps to the left front (force on the ulnar edge of the palm) when the left foot advances. The eyes watch the left hand, as shown in Figure 3-10.

10) Then, the right foot steps straight ahead on the circle so that the body in effect has turned to face the left side and the stance is in an

Exercises and Figures

outward or complex splay-foot. As the right foot is stepping forward on the circle, the right palm simultaneously penetrates forward from beneath the left elbow and forearm, with the palm and fingers pointing forward and the thumb curved slightly. The left palm also turns inward at the same time, the wrist turning down resulting in a standing palm below the right elbow. At this moment, the face and chest are facing the opposite direction of the original left millstone pushing gesture, as shown in Figure 3-11.

11) Then, the right palm follows the right turning waist to move upward to the right and curving slightly downward to drop on the right side. The left palm also follows the waist turning slightly inward to stop near the medial side of the right elbow, the eyes look at the right palm to form the right millstone pushing gesture, as shown in Figure 3-12.

Main Points

1) The whole body rotating palm is composed of the body rotating double knocking, body rotating double pressing and bilateral shielding hands. All the movements in the body rotating and footwork must be distinctive, stable and firm.

2) In the double knocking palm, it is necessary to sink the shoulders and drop the elbows. The point of force of the two palms are in the palm center and root. The movements in knocking palm, pushing palm, pressing palm and shielding hands must be in coordination.

3) The bilateral shielding hands are supposed to draw three circles continuously in the front of the chest. The movements of the two hands in shielding, blocking, pushing and grasping should be in coordination with the foot, hand, body and gesture.

4) The movements should be carried out skillfully. Please refer to the related parts of the first palm for the rest of the information (i.e. chicken leg, dragon body, etc.)

Liang Zhen Pu Eight Diagram Palm

Figure 3-1

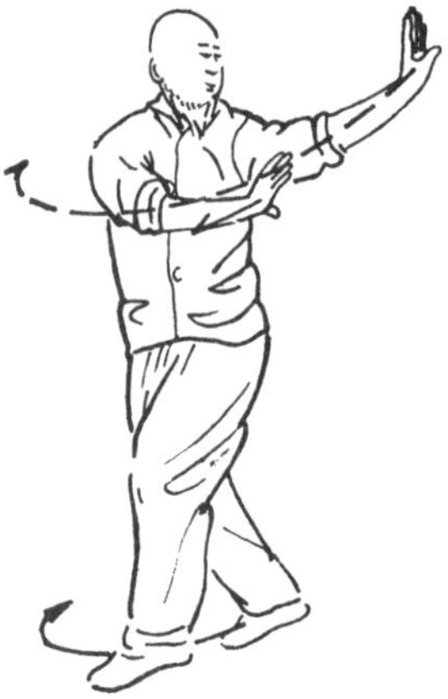

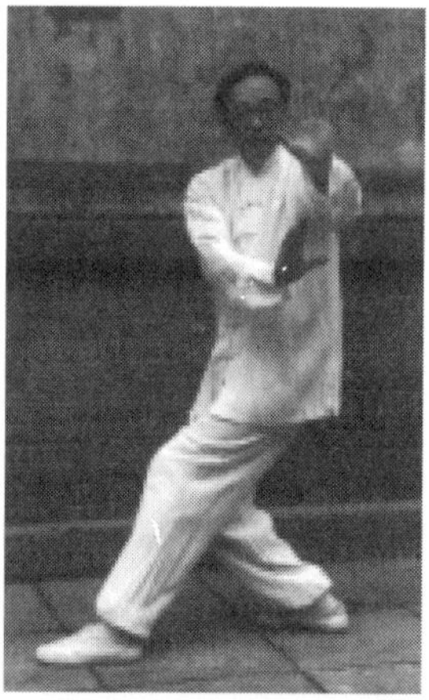

Figure 3-2

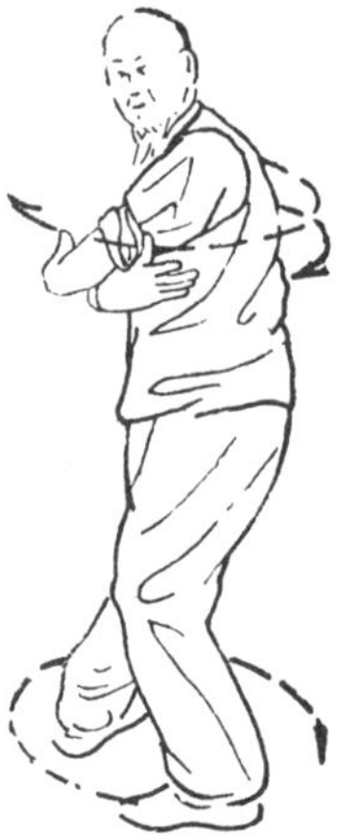

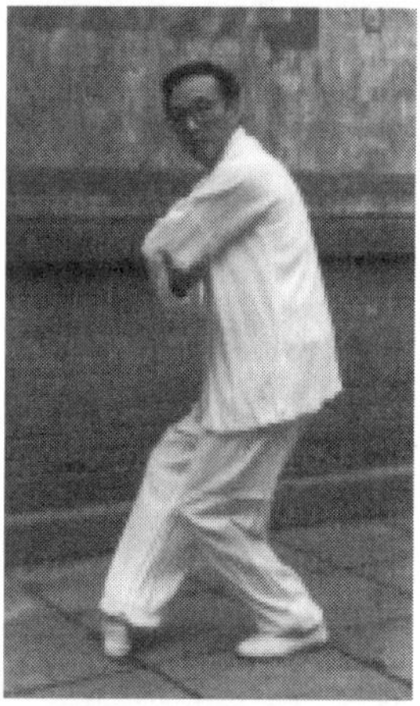

Figure 3-3

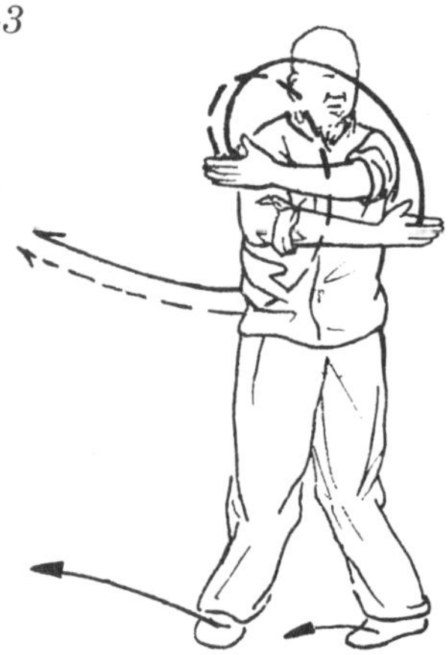

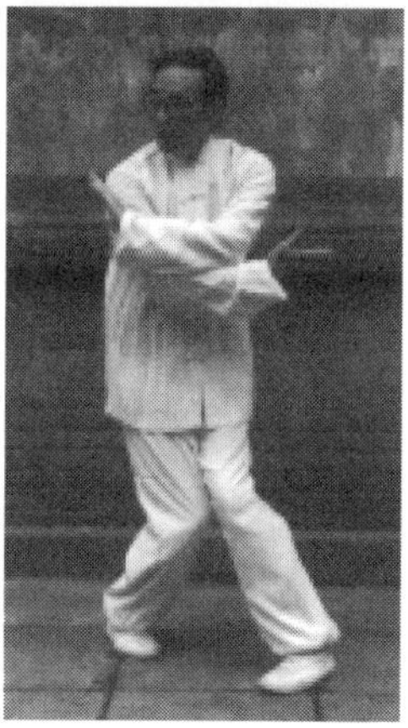

Exercises and Figures

Figure 3-4

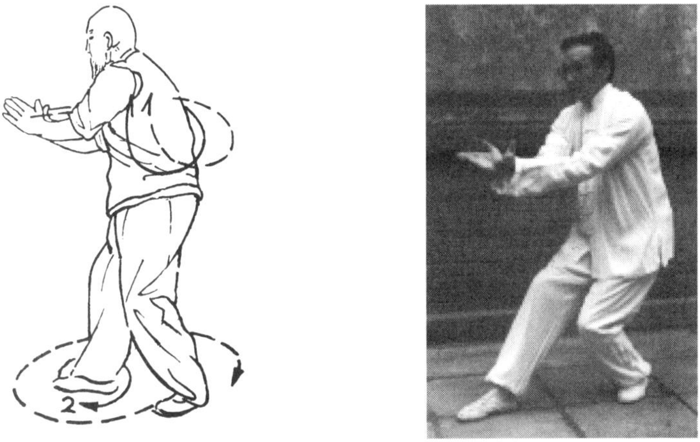

Figure 3-5

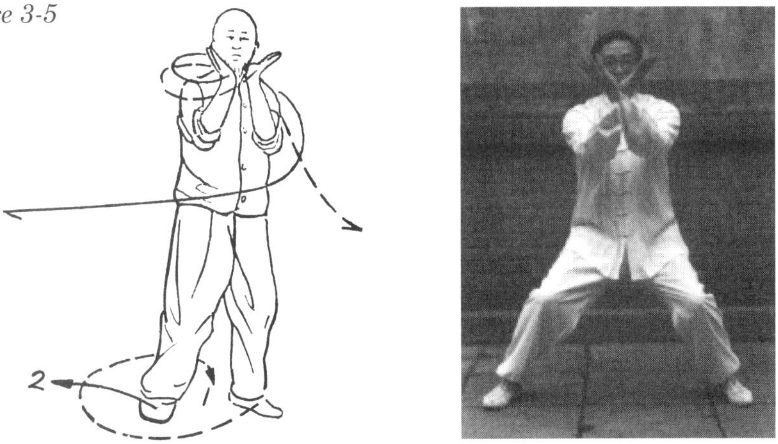

Figure 3-6

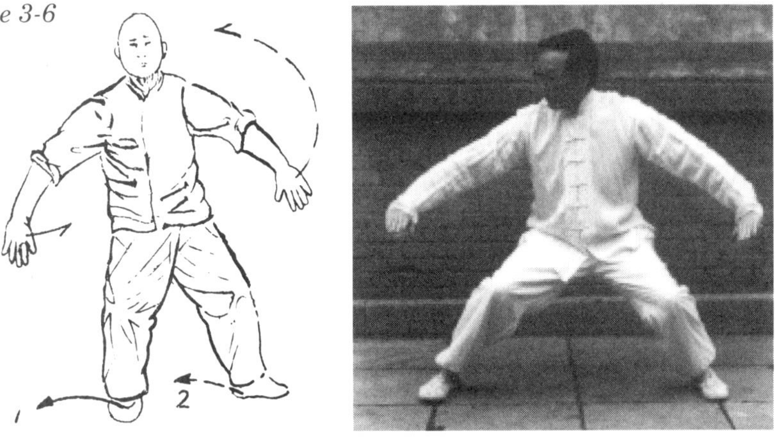

125

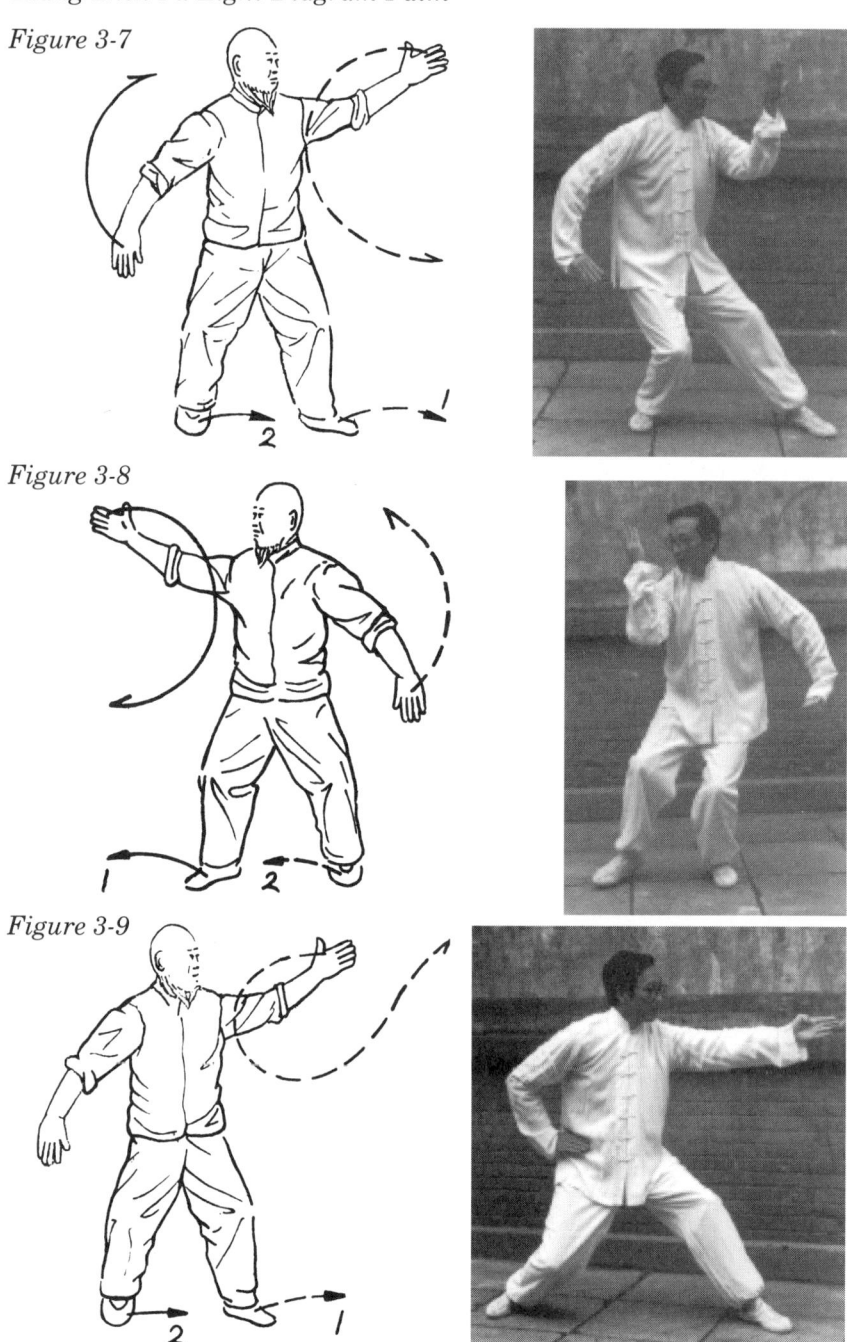

Liang Zhen Pu Eight Diagram Palm

Figure 3-7

Figure 3-8

Figure 3-9

126

Exercises and Figures

Figure 3-10

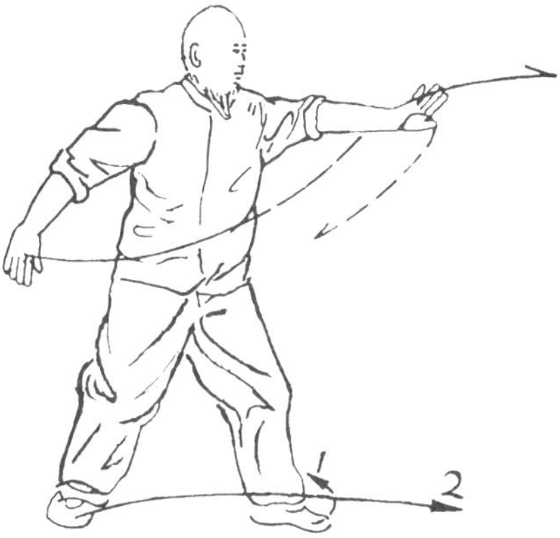

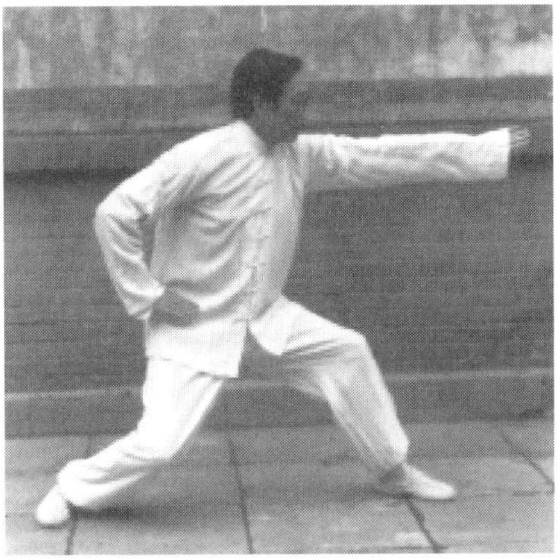

Figure 3-11

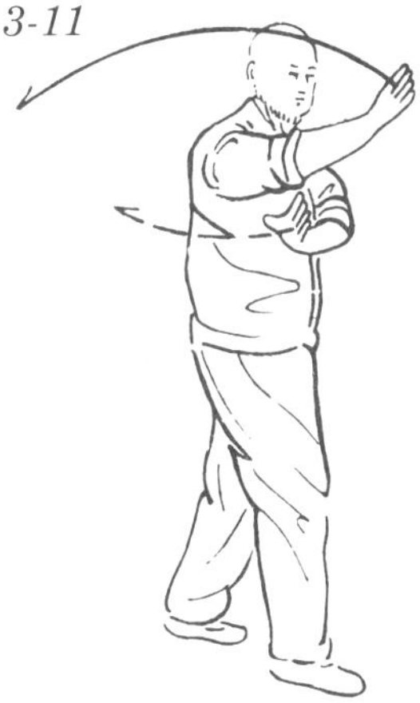

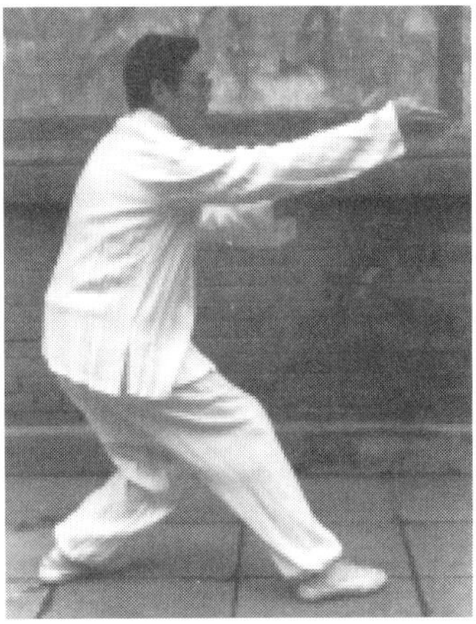

Figure 3-12

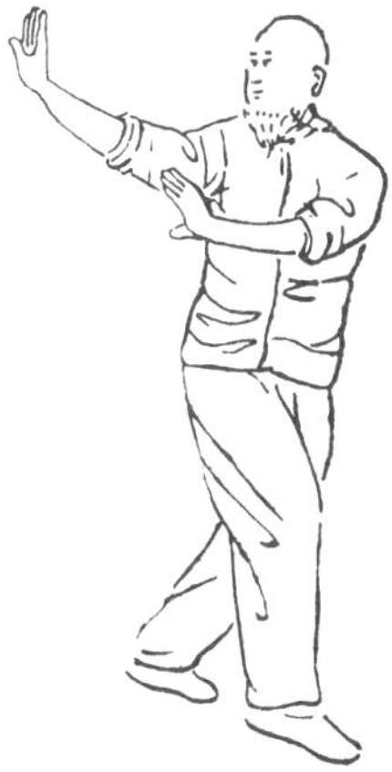

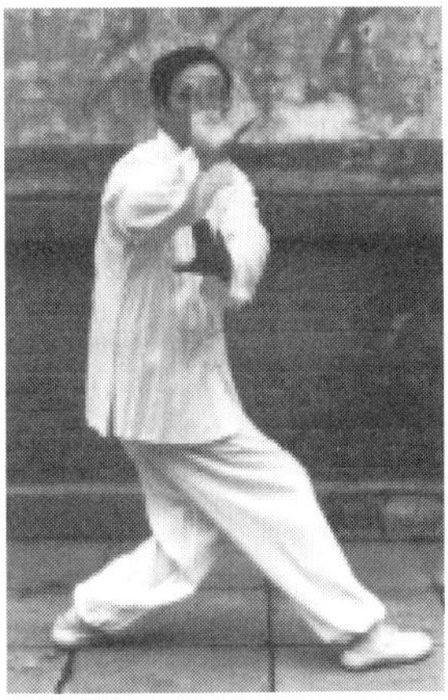

Liang Zhen Pu Eight Diagram Palm

Section 4 - Hand Chopping Palm

Movement Explanation

1) The Hand Chopping Palm, i.e. the Windmill Palm, rotates and moves to the left from the left millstone pushing gesture, as shown in Figure 4-1.

2) Walking counter clockwise, the upper body turns to the left and the gesture does not change. The right foot advances one step along the circle line and hooks the foot tip inward in a splay-foot, then the body turns to the left and the left palm supinates outward with the palm center upward, and transversely wave the radial edge to the left posterior direction. At the same time, the right palm also slightly supinates outward to have the palm center up and the eyes watching the left hand, as shown in Figure 4-2.

3) Then, the right foot does not move. The left foot swings outward and the body turns to the left. Then the right foot advances one step along the circle line. At the same time, the right palm penetrates out forward and upward underneath the left elbow and forearm, with the palm and fingers forward in a standing palm. The left palm pronates inward and sinks the wrist downward simultaneously pulling in near the lower part of the right elbow in a standing palm. At this moment, the face and chest are opposite the direction of the original left millstone pushing gesture, as shown in Figure 4-3.

4) Then the right foot hooks inward, the left foot steps around behind on the circle and the body turns backward to the left 180°. At the same time, the left hand follows the turning body to extend the palm in a high chop, either straight ahead, behind, left, or right. While hooking the right foot, the right hand moves downward to the right hip and then up to set in the front of the left side of the chest by following the body turning and palm chopping gestures, the eyes watch the left palm, as shown in Figure 4-4.

5) Then, the left foot advances a little bit swinging outward and the body turns to the left. Then the right foot advances one step along the circle line while the right palm penetrates out forward and upward underneath the left elbow and forearm, with the palm and fingers forward in a standing palm. The left palm pronates inward and sinking the wrist downward simultaneously pulls in near the lower part of the right elbow in a standing palm. At this moment, the face and chest are

Exercises and Figures

opposite the direction of the original left millstone pushing gesture, as shown in figure 4-5. (Note: The illustrator's and photographer's angle in Figure 4-5 is shot from the east, unlike the other illustrations and photos which are shot from the south. The three repetitions of the movement in this palm bring the practitioner to the eastern side of the circle. In this illustration and photo the circle is behind the practitioner.)

6) Then, the right foot hooks inward, the left foot steps around behind on the circle and the body turns backward to the left 180°. At the same time, the left hand follows the turning body to extend the palm in a high chop, either straight ahead, behind, left or right. While hooking the right foot, the right hand moves downward to the right hip and then up to set in front of the left side of the chest by following the body turning and palm chopping gestures, the eyes watch the left palm, as shown in Figure 4-6.

7) Then, the left foot advances a little bit and swings outwards and the body turns to the left. Then the right foot advances one step along the circle line. At the same time, the right palm penetrates out forward and upward underneath the left elbow and forearm, with the palm and fingers forward in a standing palm. And the left palm pronates inward and sinking the wrist downward simultaneously pulls in near the lower part of the right elbow in a standing palm. At this moment, the face and chest are opposite the direction of the original left millstone pushing gesture, as shown in Figure 4-7.

8) Then the right foot hooks inward, the left foot steps around behind on the circle and the body turns backwards to the left 180°. At the same time, the left hand follows the turning body to extend the palm in a high chop, either straight ahead, behind, left, or right. In hooking the right foot, the right hand moves downward to the right hip and then up to set in the front of the left side of the chest by following the body turning and palm chopping gestures, the eyes watching the left palm, as shown in Figure 4-8.

9) Then, the left foot advances a little bit and swings outward and the body turns to the left. Then the right foot advances one step along the circle line. At the same time, the right palm penetrates out forward and upward underneath the left elbow and forearm, with the palm and fingers forward in a standing palm. The left palm pronates inward and sinking the wrist downward simultaneously pulls in near the lower part of the right elbow in a standing palm. At this moment, the face and chest are opposite the direction of the original left millstone pushing gesture, as shown in Figure 4-9.

10) After the above continuous three chops and three palm

Liang Zhen Pu Eight Diagram Palm

penetrations, the right palm follows the right turning waist to move upwards to the right and curving slightly downward to drop on the right side. The left palm also follows the waist turning slightly inward and to stop near the medial side of the right elbow, the eyes look at the right palm to form the right millstone pushing gesture, as shown in Figure 4-10.

Main Points

1) In advancing the step, penetrating the palm and chopping the palm in turning the body, it is necessary to have the hand and foot arrive simultaneously, and to have the movements in coordination.

2) The steps advancing and retreating must be along the circle line and cannot be off of the circle line.

3) In chopping the palm, the arm must be round and flexed and cannot be extended straight. It is required to sink the shoulder and elbow. The point of force is the ulnar edge of the palm, the chopping hand and the penetrating hand should strike the level of the nose.

4) For the other requirements of the body shape, please refer to the related part of the first palm. (Chicken leg, dragon body, etc.)

Figure 4-1

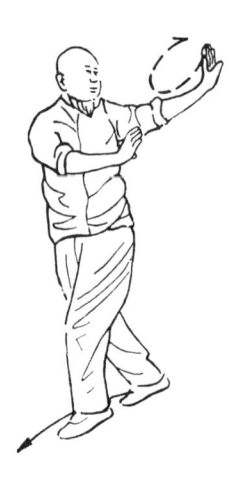

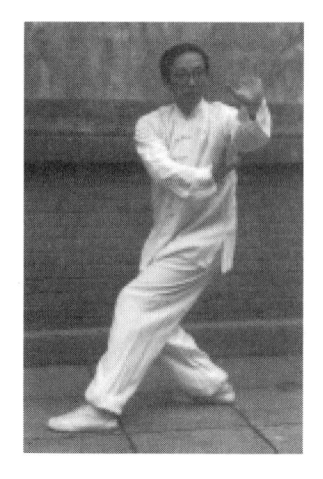

Exercises and Figures

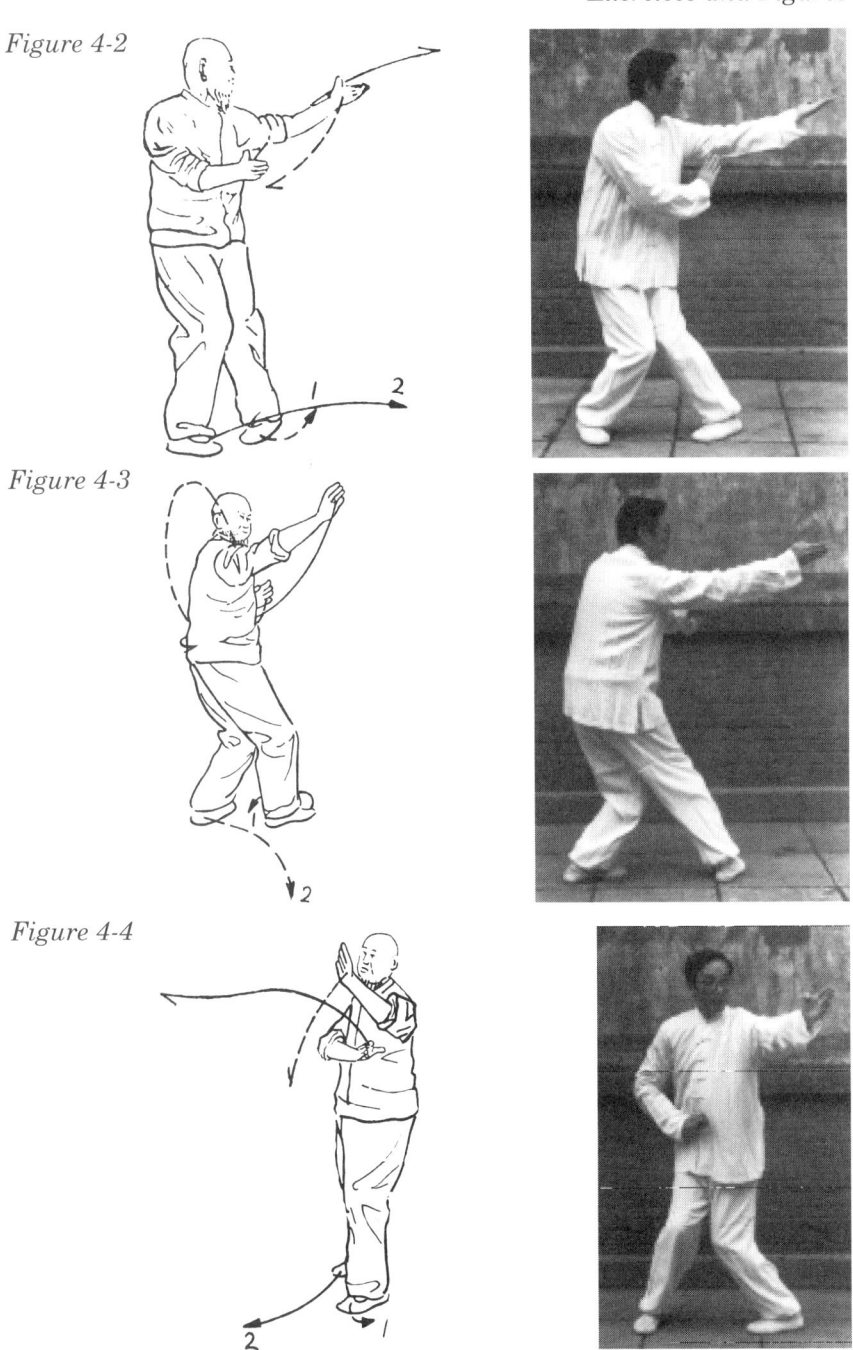

Figure 4-2

Figure 4-3

Figure 4-4

131

Liang Zhen Pu Eight Diagram Palm

Figure 4-5

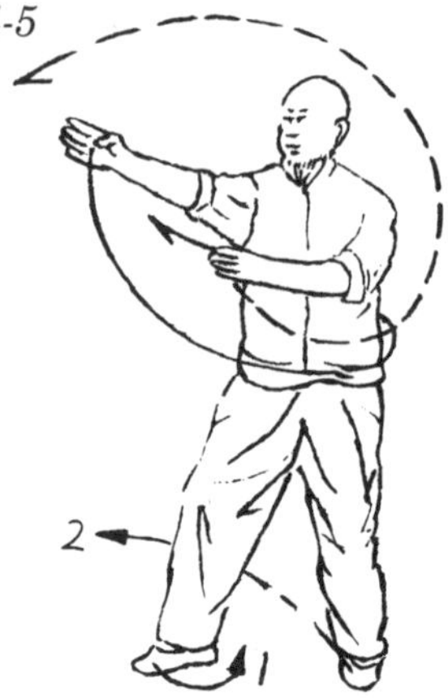

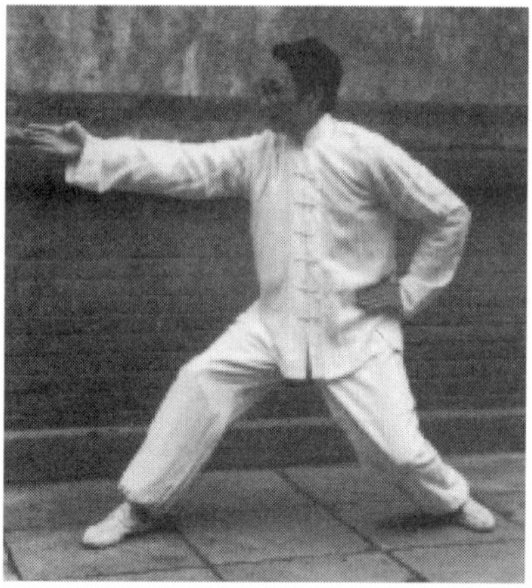

Figure 4-6

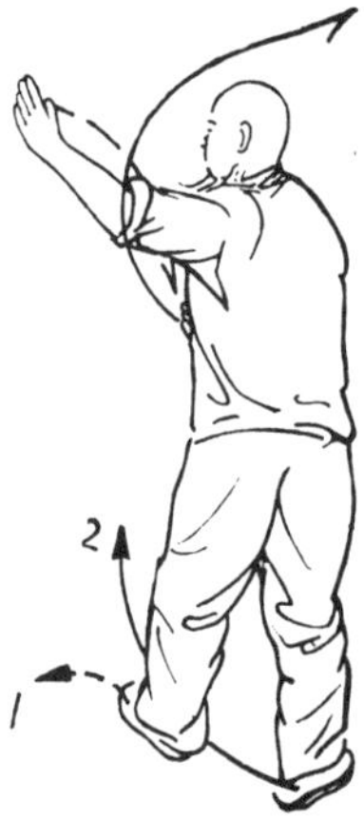

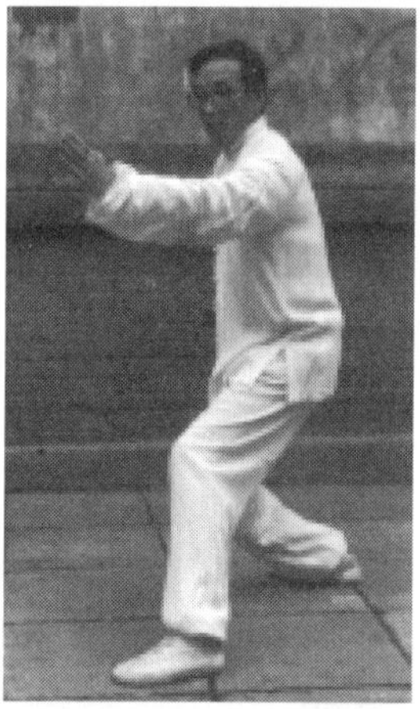

Figure 4-7

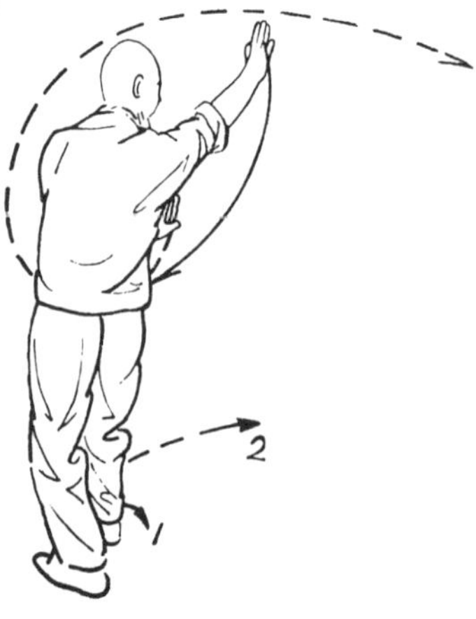

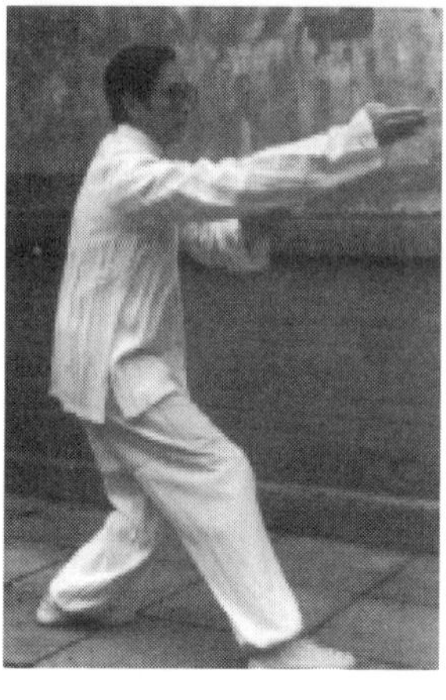

Exercises and Figures

Figure 4-8

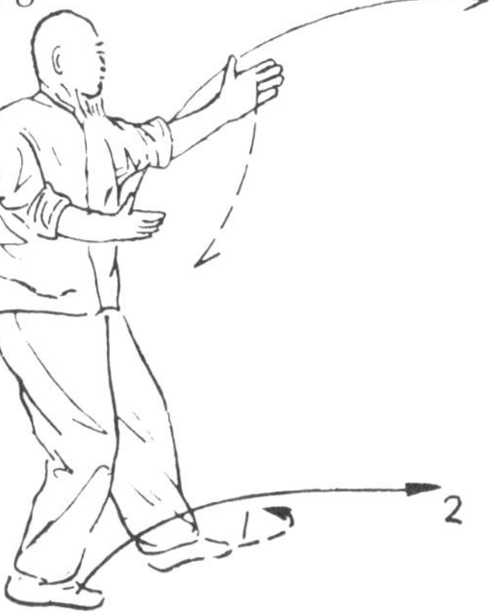

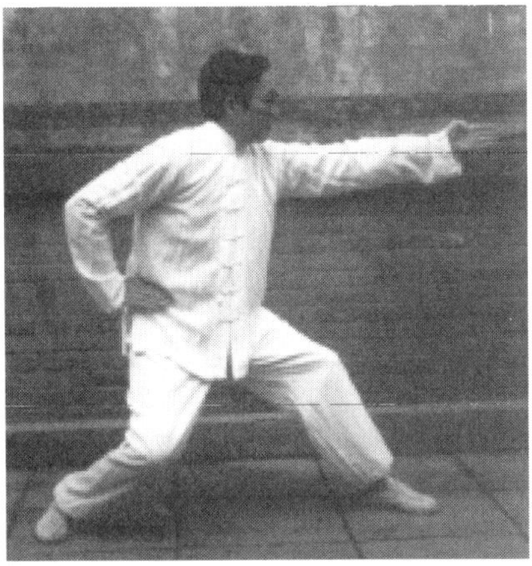

Figure 4-9

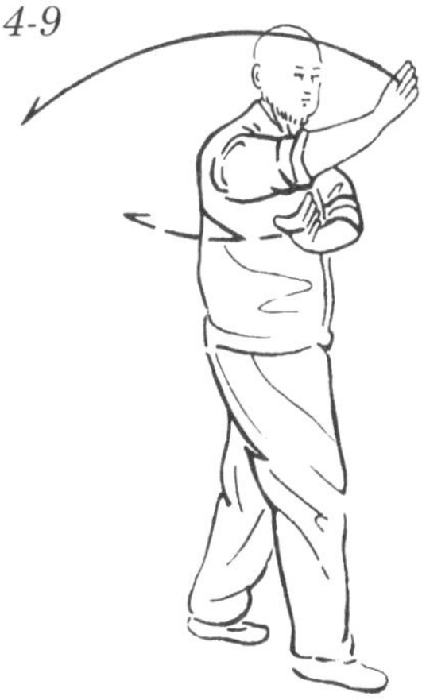

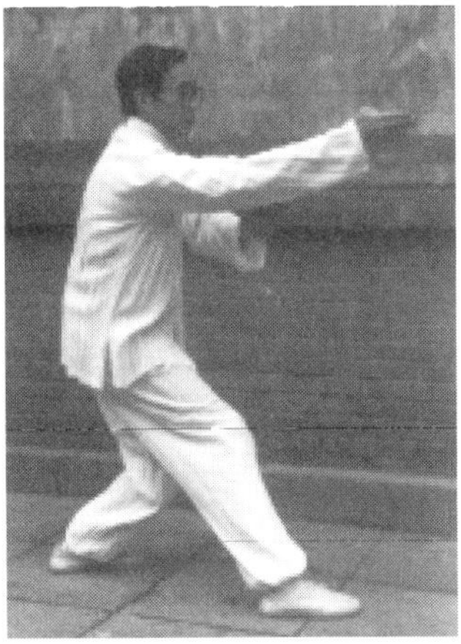

Figure 4-10

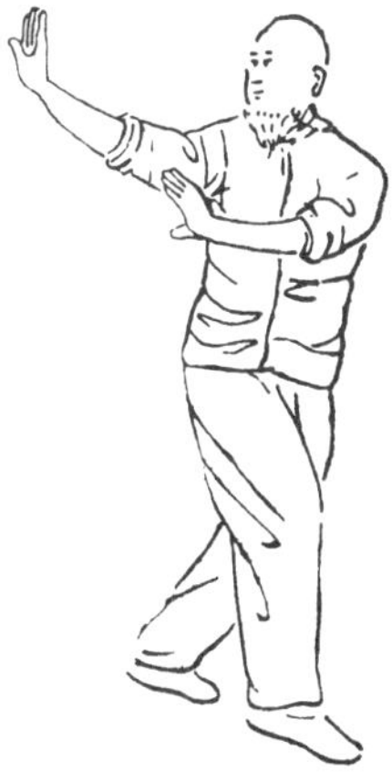

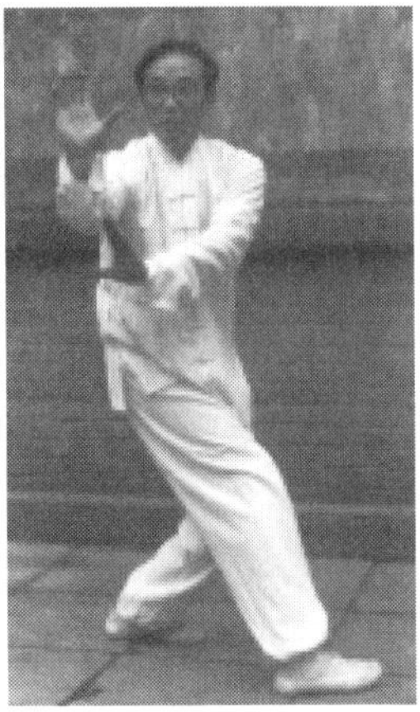

133

Liang Zhen Pu Eight Diagram Palm

Section 5 - Gesture Following Palm

Movement Explanation

1) The Gesture Following Palm rotates and moves to the left from the left millstone pushing gesture, as shown in Figure 5-1.

2) The right foot advances one step on the circle, with the foot tip hooked inwards in a normal splay-foot. Then the body turns to the left, the left palm supinates outward with the palm up and moving to the posterior left leading with the radial side of the wrist. At the same time, the right palm also rotates outward for having the palm upward, the eyes watching the left hand, as shown in Figure 5-2.

3) Then, the left foot moves forward slightly, the right foot advances one big step on the circle, the weight shifting to the right leg, the knees bent and body lowered. The left foot hangs over the right foot and steps into a right legged stance for the upper palm penetration (also possible to use the right bow stance for the upper palm penetration). While stepping with the right foot, the left palm rotates inward and strikes downward (with the palm center downward) while the right palm penetrates out upward underneath the left hand (with the palm center toward your own face but above the head), the eyes watch the right palm, as shown in Figure 5-3.

4) Then, the left foot draws back slightly with the toe on the ground, the right foot hooks inward and the left foot takes one big step back on the circle, turn to the left rear (facing the circle), lowering the body with the weight on the right foot in a right sweeping step. The right palm does not change while the left palm thrusts downward following the left foot (the left palm pronates inward as much as possible so that the palm center is up) extending and spreading to the left, as shown in Figure 5-4.

5) The weight then gradually shifts to the left leg in a bow stance. While shifting the weight, the left hand supinates outward 360° so that as the palm turns forward it ends with the palm center up and the right palm follows to rotate inwards in 360° placing the palm center upward in a reverse position. Both palms extend and spread flatly. The eyes watch the left hand, as shown in Figure 5-5.

6) Then the weight shifts to the right leg in a right bow stance, and both palms move simultaneously, that is, the right palm supinates

Exercises and Figures

outwards (360°), the left palm pronates inwards (360°) to have the right palm upward and the left palm upward as well, both hands extend and spreading flatly with the eyes watching the right palm, as shown in Figure 5-6.

7) Then, the weight shifts to the left leg in a left bow stance, and again both palms move simultaneously, that is, the left palm supinates outward (360 °), the right palm pronates inward (360°), to have the left palm upwards and the right palm upward as well, both hands extending and spreading flatly with the eyes watching the left palm, as shown in Figure 5-7.

8) Following the above movement of the left bow step gesture, the left foot swings slightly outward, the right foot advances one step on the circle. At the same time, the right palm penetrates out forward and upward underneath the left elbow and forearm, with the palm and fingers forward in a standing palm. The left palm pronates inward and sinking the wrist downward simultaneously pulls in near the lower part of the right elbow in a standing palm. At this movement, the face and chest are opposite the direction of the original left millstone pushing gesture, as shown in Figure 5-8.

9) Then the right palm follows the right turning waist to move upward to the right and curving slightly downward to drop on the right side (the palm facing the center of the circle with the shoulder, elbow and wrist sunken downward and the finger tip at the level of the eyebrow). The left palm also follows the waist turning slightly inward to stop near the medial side of the right elbow (the palm faces to the circle center obliquely), the eyes look at the right palm to form the right millstone pushing gesture, as shown in Figure 5-9.

Main Points

1) It is required to lift the sacrum throughout the whole series of movements and to be in coordination when the weight moves laterally.

2) It is mandatory to integrate the waist and leg force to rotate, extend and spread the arms bilaterally. It is also important to maintain the shoulder and elbow sunken when the arms extend almost straight.

3) For the other requirements of the body shape, please refer to the related part of the first palm.

Liang Zhen Pu Eight Diagram Palm

Figure 5-1

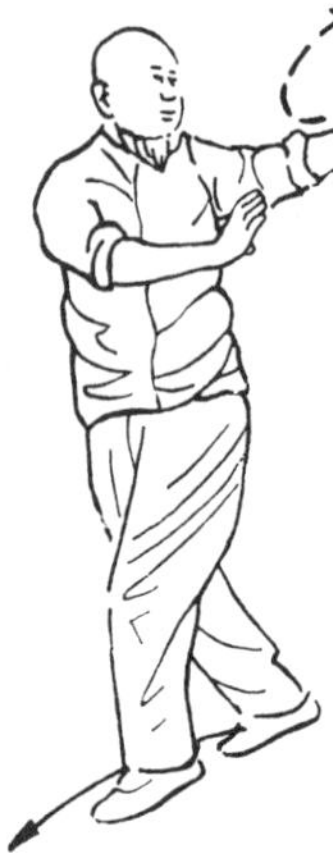

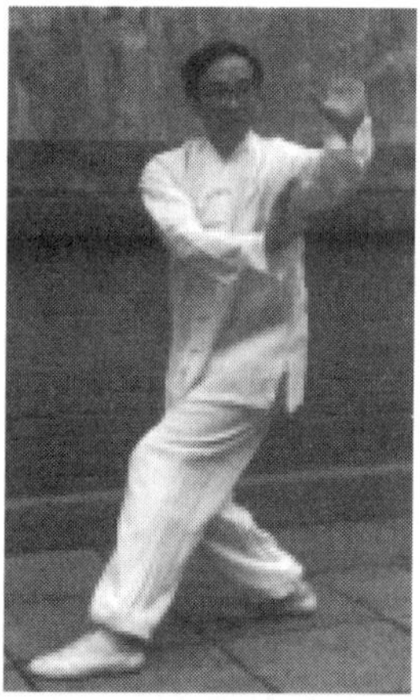

Figure 5-2

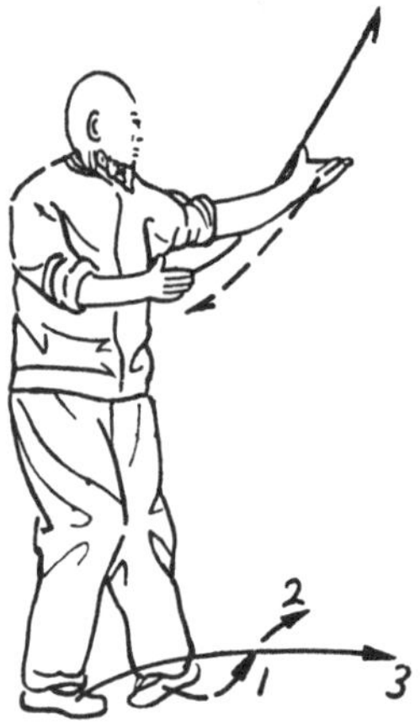

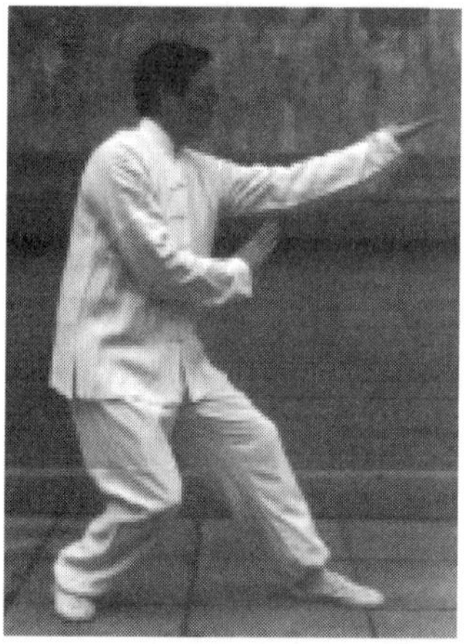

Figure 5-3

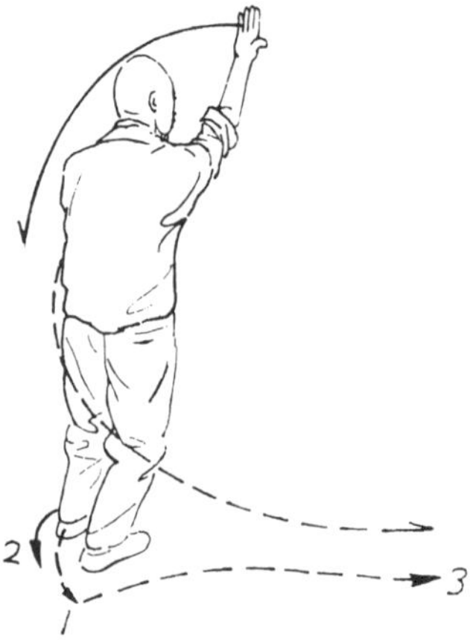

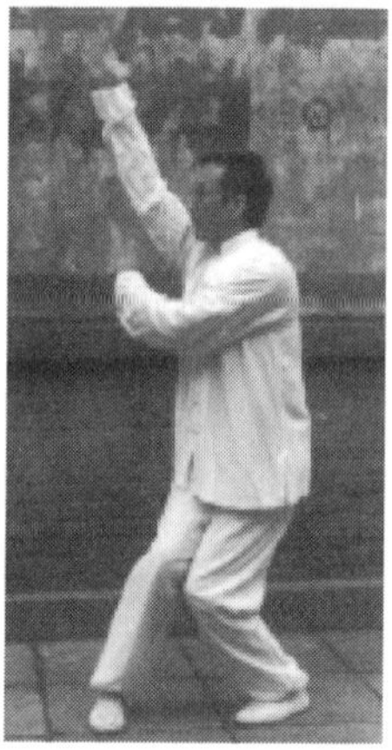

136

Exercises and Figures

Figure 5-4

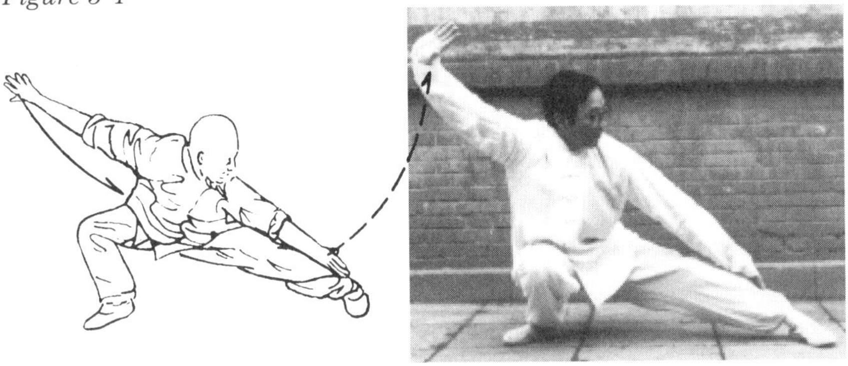

Figure 5-5

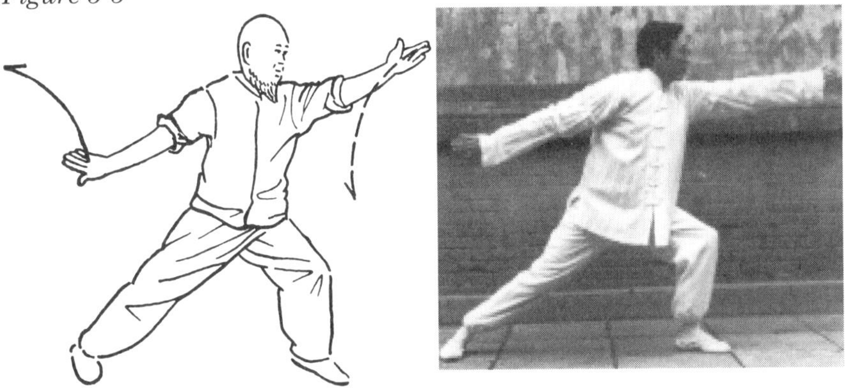

Figure 5-6

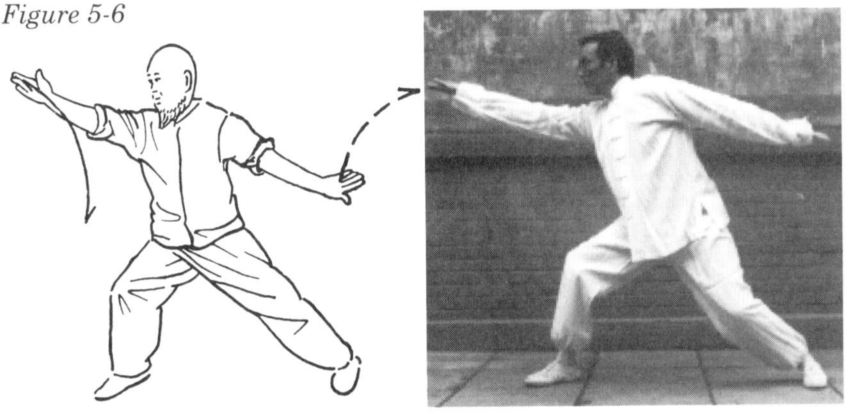

Liang Zhen Pu Eight Diagram Palm

Figure 5-7

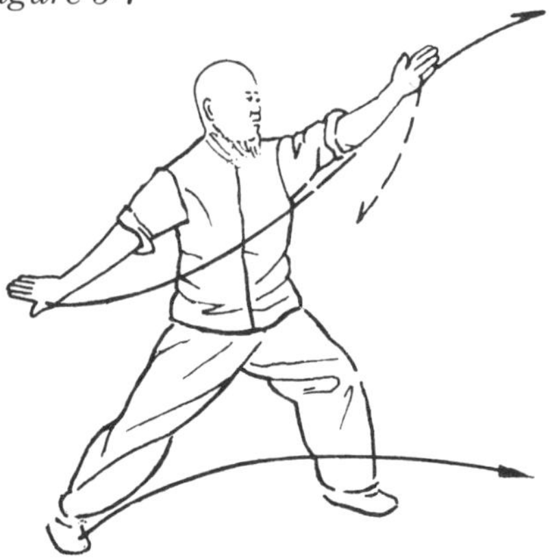

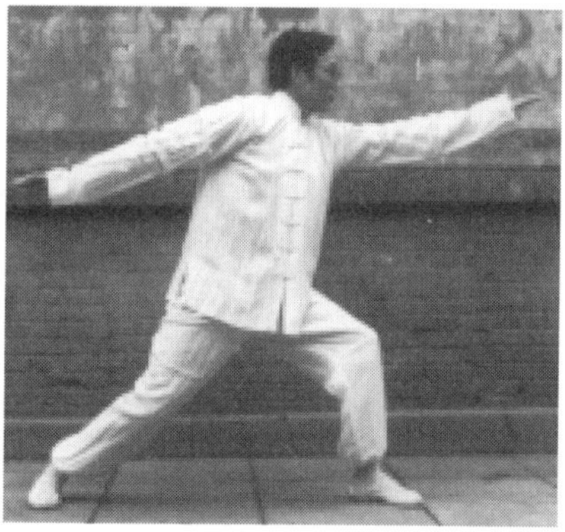

Figure 5-8

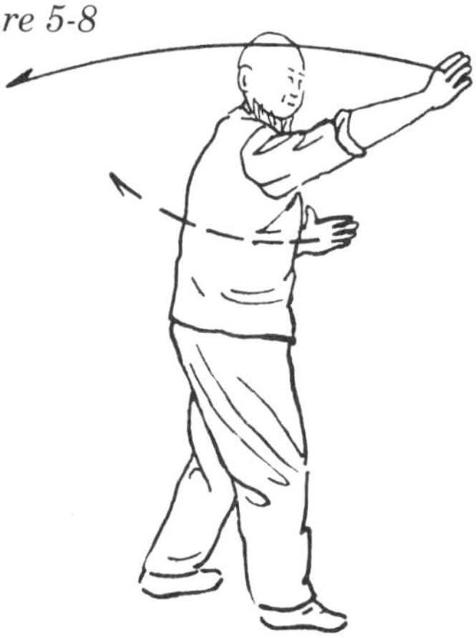

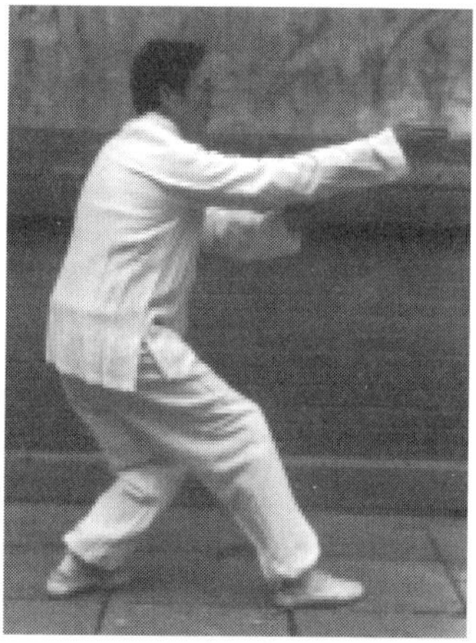

Figure 5-9

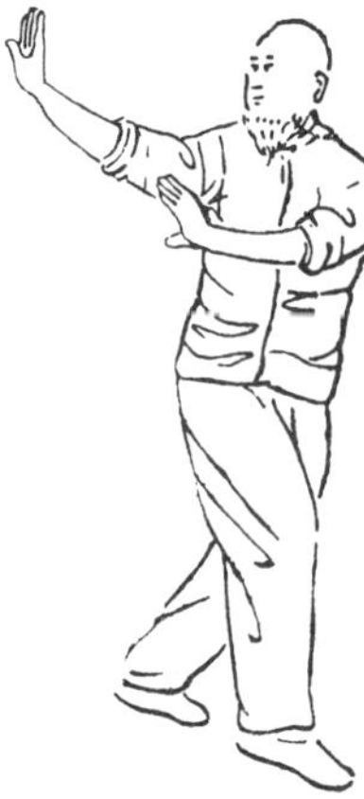

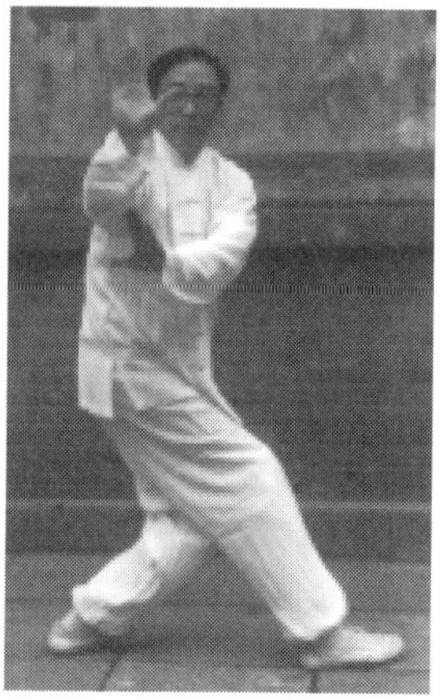

Exercises and Figures

Section 6 - Step Following Palm

Movement Explanation

1) The Step Following Palm rotates and moves to the left from the left millstone pushing gesture, as shown in Figure 6-1.

2) From the left millstone pushing posture, the right foot advances one step along the circle line with the foot tip hooked inward in a splayfoot. Then the body turns to the left, the left palm rotates outward to have the palm center upward, after which the radial side of the wrist moves transversely to the left posterior. At the same time, the right palm also rotates outward to have the palm center upward, the eyes watching the left palm, as shown in Figure 6-2.

3) Without moving the upper body, the left foot swings outward and the body turns to the left. Then the right foot advances one step along the circle line. At the same time, the right palm penetrates out forward and upward underneath the left elbow and forearm, with the palm and fingers forward in a standing palm. The left palm pronates inward and sinking the wrist downward simultaneously pulls in near the lower part of the right elbow in a standing palm. At this moment, the face and chest are opposite the direction of the original left millstone pushing gesture, as shown in Figure 6-3.

4) After toeing the right foot in, the left foot steps backward one big step to the left posterior on the circle (northeast to east), the body turns to the right and squats in a low half horse step. At the same time, the right palm rotates outward in a small circle supinating in a hooking and gripping action. Then following the body turning gesture, both hands in fists pull down to the dorsum of the right foot, and the eyes watching the hands, as shown in Figure 6-4.

5) The waist turns to the left and the weight shifts to the left leg, both hands gripping in a left bow stance, as shown in Figure 6-5.

6) Then the right foot advances one step in a chicken leg step gesture. While turning the waist to the left, the two hands lift to the front of the lower abdomen to inscribe an arc first to the left, then upward and over to the right (ending with the palm toward the center of the circle) in a right millstone pushing gesture, as shown in Figure 6-6.

Liang Zhen Pu Eight Diagram Palm

Main Points

1) It is required that the hands rub the body to follow the backward turning and body turning gestures.
2) Backward turning and body turning movements in turning the body to pull downward will be effective only when the hands, body and footwork are in coordination.
3) Please refer to the related parts of the first palm for the other information.

Figure 6-1

Figure 6-2

Exercises and Figures

Figure 6-3

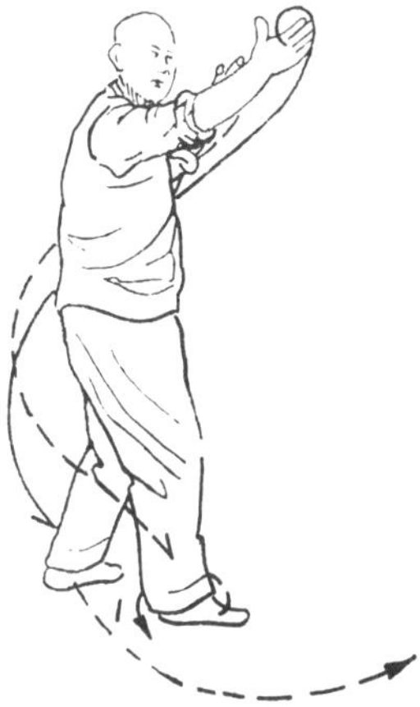

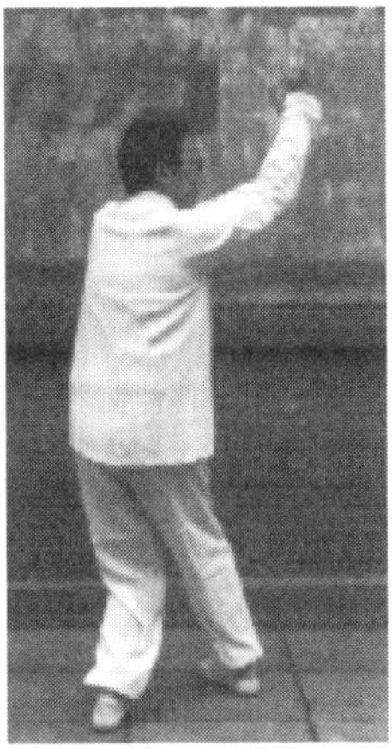

Figure 6-4

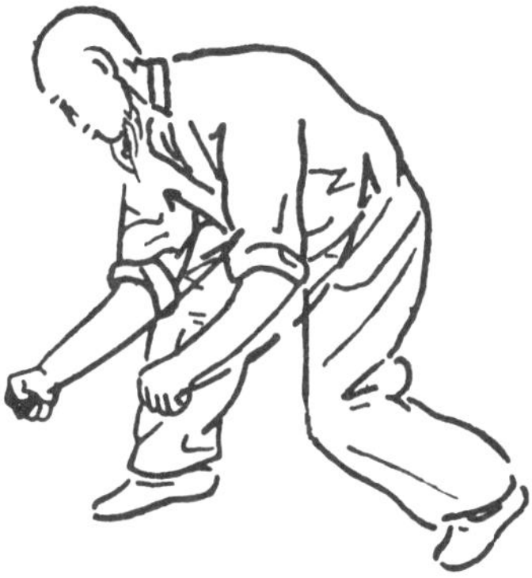

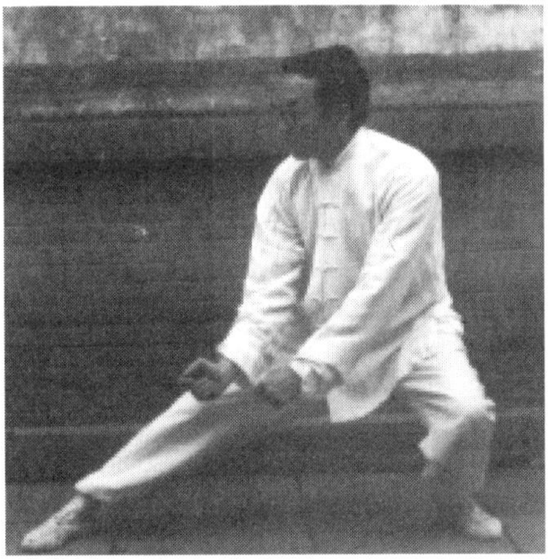

Figure 6-5

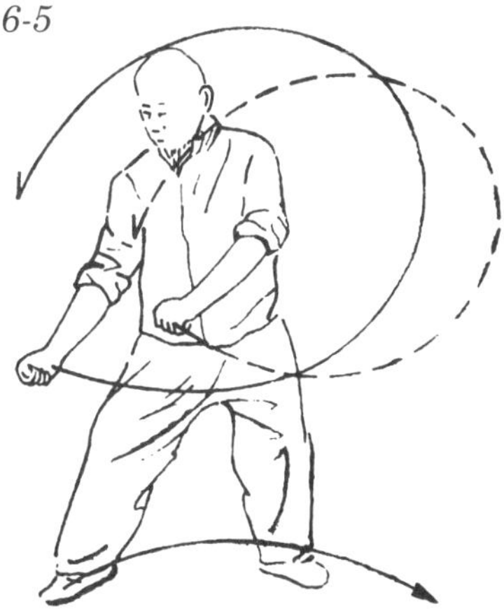

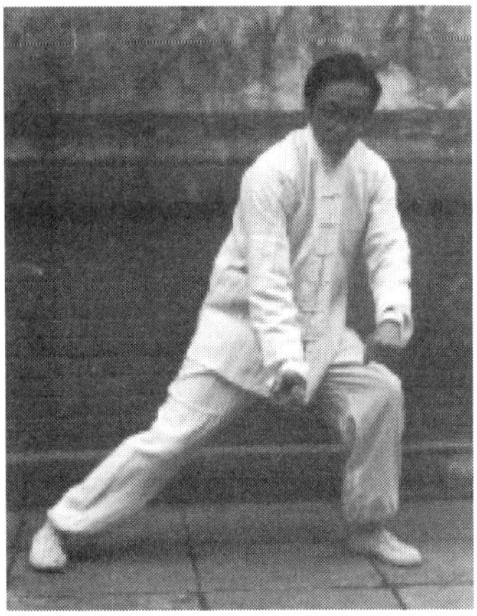

141

Liang Zhen Pu Eight Diagram Palm

Figure 6-6

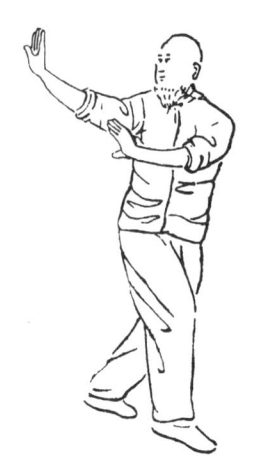

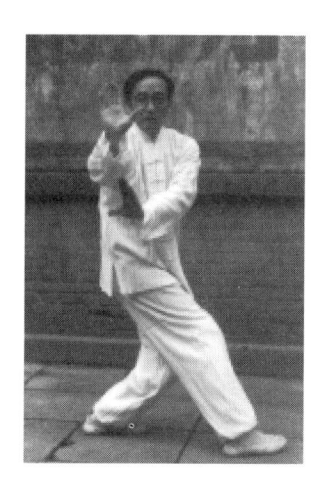

Section 7 - Downward Dropping Palm

Movement Explanation

1) This palm starts as shown in Figure 7-1.
2) The right foot advances one step on the circle, with the foot hooking inward in a normal splay-foot. The waist turns to the left to face the circle, then both palms first supinate then the right immediately pronates to have the palm center upward, the right palm positioned under the left elbow, as shown in Figure 7-2.
3) Continuing the above movement, the body turns to the left, the left foot swings outward and the right hand does not move. When the left foot moves outward, the left palm first supinates outward (with the palm upward), and then pronates to the underneath of the left armpit (the palm faces upward and the thumb moves inward to point to the left), as shown in Figure 7-3.
4) When the left palm rotates in front of the left hip, the right foot steps around and behind the left side of the left foot, with the foot turned inward as much as possible in a complex splay-foot, and then the waist follows turning to the left (at this moment, the back faces to the circle center). The left palm continues supinating to push upward (the palm center is still upward, the thumb point to the left and the other fingers point outwards). At the same time, the weight stays on the right leg, and the right palm (upward) penetrates out from underneath the left armpit.

Exercises and Figures

Then the waist turns to the left, the left elbow lifts upward and the head goes out under the left elbow. The left palm (upward) spirals upward, posteriorly, over the head and to the left, and then faces the circle, as shown Figure 7-4.

5) Then, both palms extend and spread to their respective sides flatly (with the palms up). In the moment of extending and spreading the two palms, the left foot moves slightly forward and the body sinks, as shown in Figure 7-5.

6) Following the above movement, the body turns to the left and the left foot swings outward and the right hand does not move. When the left foot moves outward, the left palm first supinates outward (with the palm upward), and then pronates to the underneath of the left armpit (the palm faces upward and the thumb moves inward to point to the left). When the left palm rotates to the front of the left hip, the right foot steps around and behind the left side of the left foot, with the foot turned inward as much as possible in a complex splay-foot and the waist following turning to the left. At this moment, the back faces to the circle center. The left palm continues supinating to push upward (the palm center is still upward, the thumb points to the left and the other fingers point outward). At the same time, the weight stays on the right leg, and the right palm (upward) penetrates out from underneath the left armpit. Then the waist turns to the left, the left elbow lifts upward and the head goes out under the left elbow. The left palm (upward) spirals upward, posteriorly, over the head and to the left, and then faces the circle, as shown in Figure 7-6. Note 1.

7) Continuing the above movement, the body turns to the left, the left foot swings outward and the right hand does not move. When the left foot moves outward, the left palm first supinates outward (with the palm upward), and then pronates to the underneath of the left armpit (the palm faces upward and the thumb moves inward to point to the left). When the left palm rotates to the left front of the left hip, the right foot steps around and behind the left side of the left foot, with the foot turned inward as much as possible in a complex splay-foot, and then the waist follows turning to the left (at this moment, the back faces to the center of the circle). The left palm continues supinating to push upwards (the palm center is still upward, the thumb points to the left and the other fingers point outward). At the same time, the weight stays on the right leg, and the right palm (upward) penetrates out from underneath the left armpit. Then the waist turns to the left, the left elbow lifts upward and the head goes out under the left elbow. The left palm (upward) spirals upward, posteriorly, over the head and to the left, and then faces the

circle, as shown in Figure 7-7. Note 1.

8) Following the above movement, the left foot moves outward a little bit, the right foot advances one step on the circle line. At the same time, the right palm penetrates out forward and upward underneath the left elbow and forearm, with the palm and fingers forward to be a standing palm. The left palm pronates inward and sinking the wrist downwards simultaneously pulls in near the lower part of the right elbow in a standing palm. At this moment, the face and chest are opposite the direction of the original left millstone pushing gesture, as shown in Figure 7-8.

9) Then, the right palm follows the right turning waist to move upward to the right curving slightly downward to drop on the right side the palm facing the center of the circle, with the shoulder, elbow and wrist sunken downward and the finger tip at the level of the eyebrow. The left palm also follows the waist turning slightly inward to stop near the medial side of the right elbow (the palm faces to the circle center obliquely), the eyes look at the right palm to form the right millstone pushing gesture, as shown in Figure 7-9.

Main Points

1) The palm always faces upward when the left palm rotates and moves. When both arms extend and spread bilaterally, it is necessary to keep the arms round and flexed and to keep the shoulders and elbows sunken.

2) When the right foot moves around to the lateral side of the left foot, it is necessary to hook the foot inward as much as possible, the right foot curves about 270° with the knees close together.

3) The steps always move on the circle in the movements of the three rotations, arm extension and spreading.

4) In the movements, the hands, feet and body must be in coordination. Please refer to the related parts for the other requirements.

Note 1: The movement routes in Figures 7-3, 7-4 and 7-5 are the explanatory figures of the main movements in the Downward Dropping Palm which repeat themselves two more times. In order to illustrate the movement routes in their entirety, in the following Figures 7-6 and 7-7, the interim movements are not shown but are addressed in the discussion merely as a continuation to Figure 7-5.

Exercises and Figures

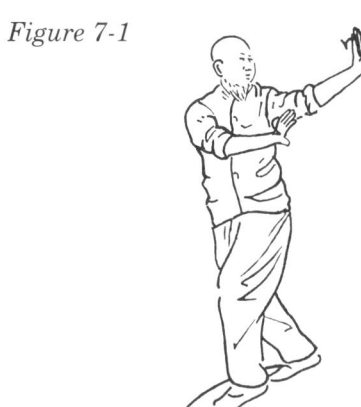

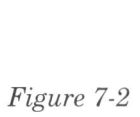

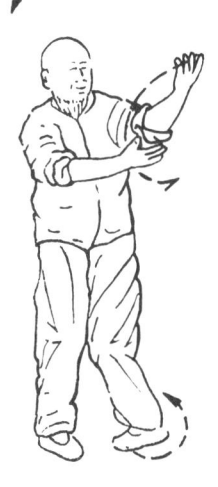

Figure 7-1

Figure 7-2

Figure 7-3

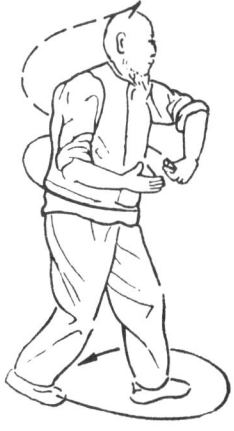

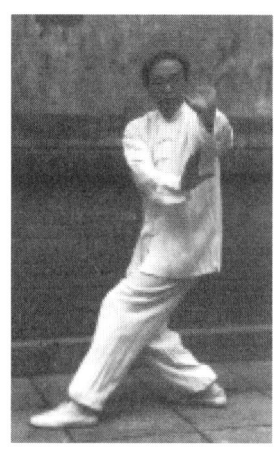

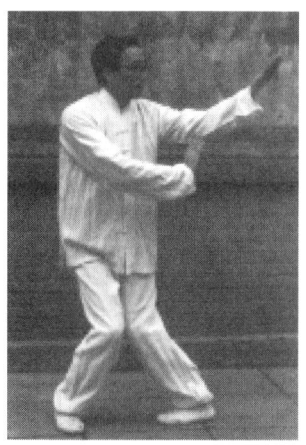

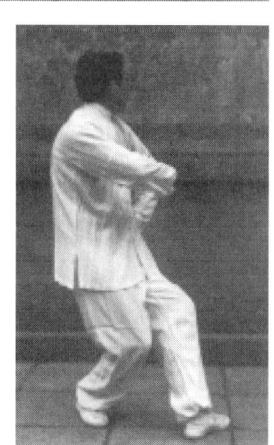

145

Liang Zhen Pu Eight Diagram Palm

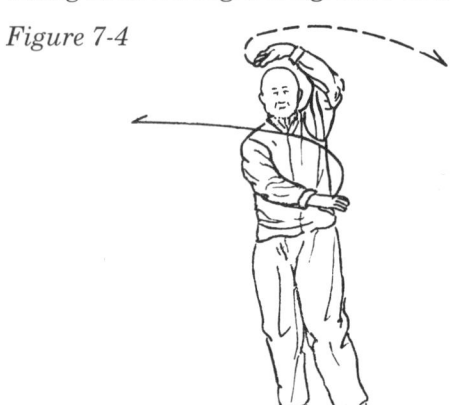

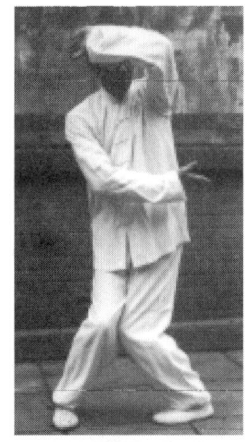

Figure 7-4

Figure 7-5

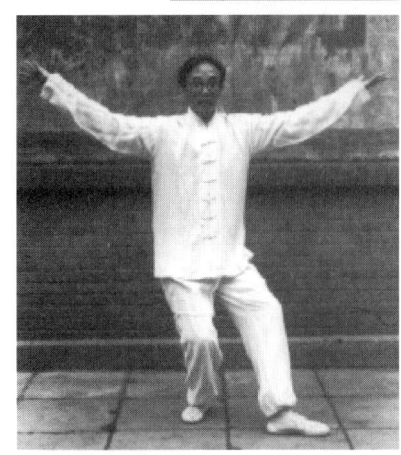

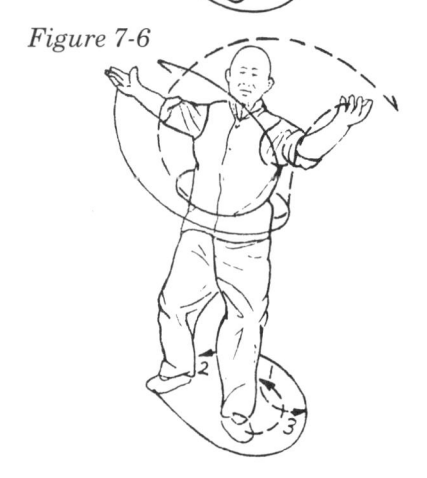

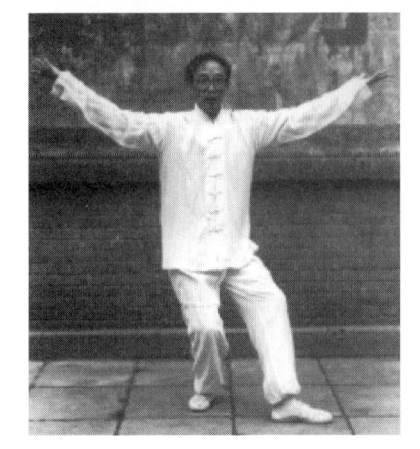

Figure 7-6

146

Exercises and Figures

Figure 7-7

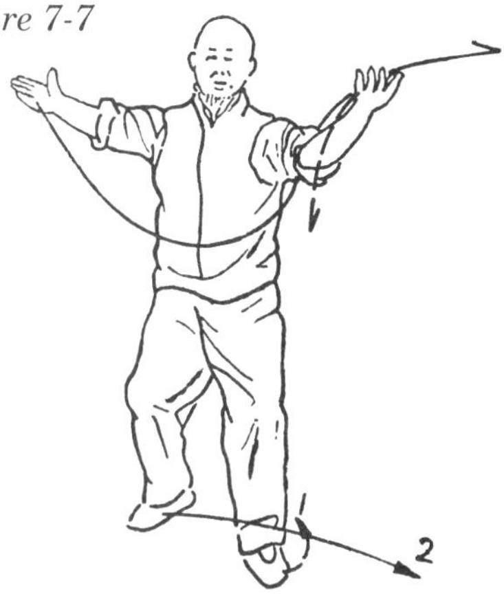

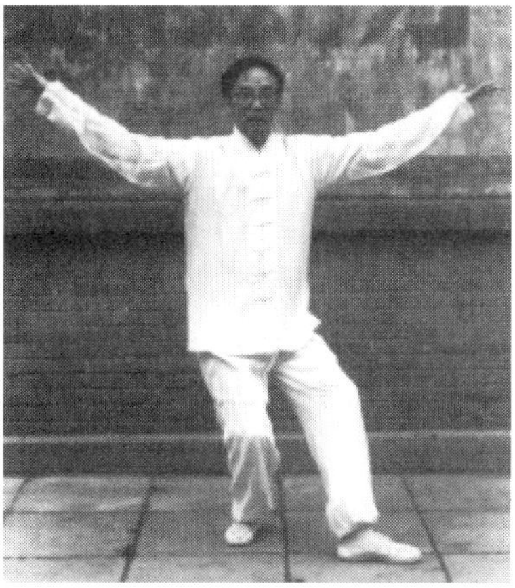

Figure 7-8

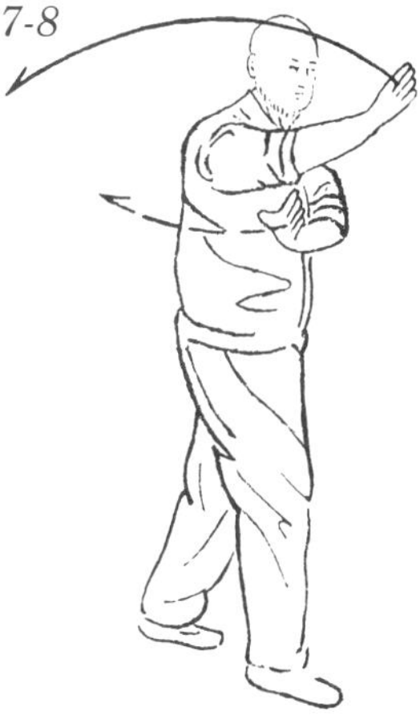

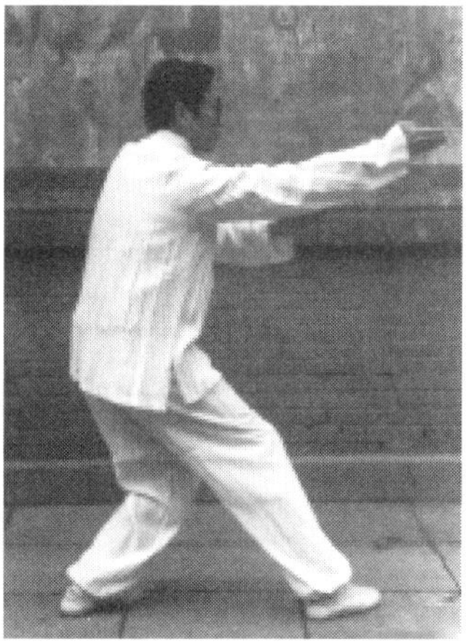

Figure 7-9

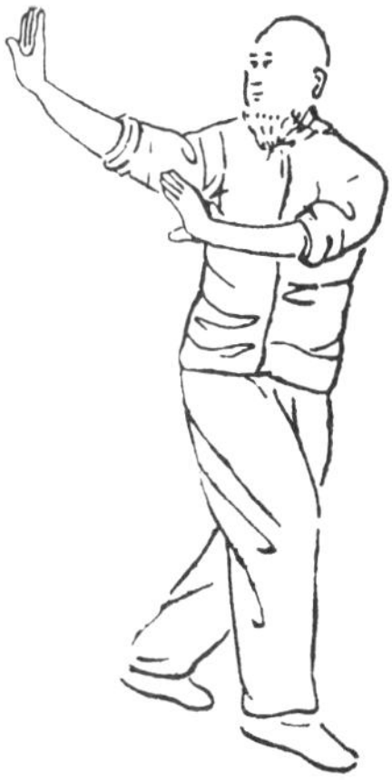

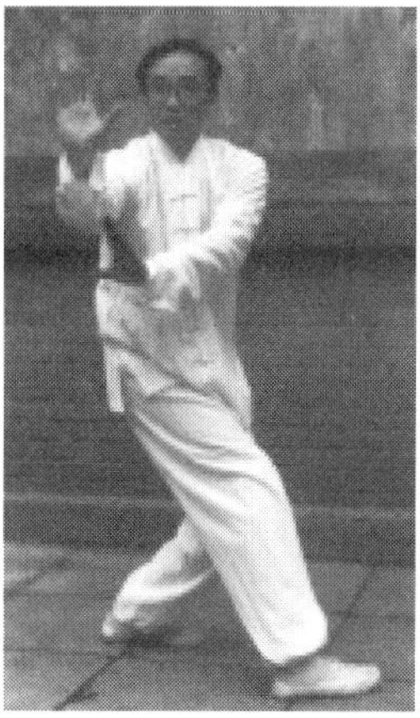

147

Liang Zhen Pu Eight Diagram Palm

Section 8 - Flat Penetrating Palm

Movement Explanation

1) This palm starts as shown in Figure 8-1.

2) The right foot advances one step on the circle and then hooks inward in a splayfoot. Then the body turns to the left, the left palm supinates outward (with the palm upward) and moves transversely to the left posterior leading with the radial side of the palm. At the same time, the right palm also slightly supinates outward to have the palm upward, the eyes watching the left hand, as shown in Figure 8-2.

3) Planting on the right foot, the left foot moves outward and the body turns to the left. Then, the right foot advances one step straightly along the circle, and at the same time, the right palm penetrates out forward underneath the left elbow and forearm (with the palm down), and the left palm also rotates inward simultaneously to turn the wrist and move downward to stop at the lower part of the right elbow in a lateral prone palm. This is the right penetrating palm gesture. The face and chest are opposite to the direction of the original left millstone pushing gesture. See Figure 8-3.

4) Then the right foot moves outward slightly and the left foot hooks one step forward on the circle. At the same time, the left palm pronely penetrates out underneath the right elbow and forearm as in the previous movement, and the right palm also simultaneously pronates inward to turn the wrist and move downward to place it at the lower part of the left elbow in a lateral prone palm. This is the left penetrating palm gesture, as shown in Figure 8-4.

5) Following the above movement, the left foot moves slightly outward and the right foot advances one step straightly on the circle. At the same time, the right palm pronely penetrates out forward and upward underneath the left elbow and forearm (with the fingers forward and the palm downward). The left palm also simultaneously pronates inward to turn the wrist and moves downward to place at the lower part of the right elbow in a lateral prone palm. This is also the right penetrating palm gesture, as shown in Figure 8-5.

6) Following the above movement, the right foot rotates inward and hooks the step as much as possible, simultaneously the right palm pronates inward and moves backward to the lateral side of the left ribs (with the palm downward), the body turns to a left posterior and the right

Exercises and Figures

foot turns in and the left foot follows the left turning body to walk one step in the left posterior direction on the circle. While turning the body and advancing the step, the right hand strikes along the abdomen low and to the left side and the left high (the point of force is on the ulnar edge of the palm) at the level of the chin, as shown in Figure 8-6.

7) Then as the right foot advances one step, the left palm rotates outward in 90° and then rotates inward to turn the wrist. And the right palm penetrates out forward underneath the left elbow and forearm in a standing palm, the left palm follows the previous movement to move downward and set in the area below the right elbow, the eyes watching the right palm, as shown in Figure 8-7.

8) Following the above movement, the waist turns to the right, the right palm follows the right turning of the waist to curve upward to the right and slightly downward, and drop on the right side (with the palm toward the circle center), with the shoulder, elbow and wrist sunken and with the finger tip at the level of the nose. The left palm also follows the turning waist to rotate inward slightly and place in near the site of the right elbow (with the palm obliquely toward the center of the circle), the eyes watch the right palm in a right millstone pushing gesture, as shown in Figure 8-8.

Main Points

1) The continuous three palm penetrations (left, right and left) are all performed on a circle. But it is not necessary to adhere to form after skillful practice and one can practice the palm penetration forward as well.

2) In the penetrating palm and the striking palm, the arm cannot extend too straight, so it is necessary to sink the shoulder and elbow and the point of force is in the finger tips.

3) All movements, such as advancing step, swinging step, penetrating palm and striking palm, must be distinctive and in coordination for skillful power release.

4) For other requirements, please refer to the related parts in the first palm.

Liang Zhen Pu Eight Diagram Palm

Figure 8-1

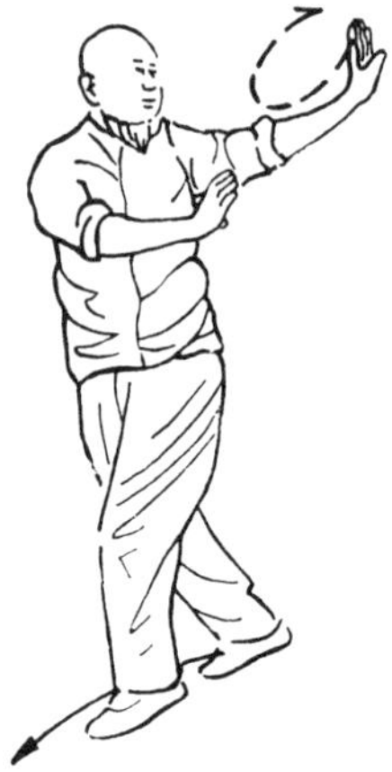

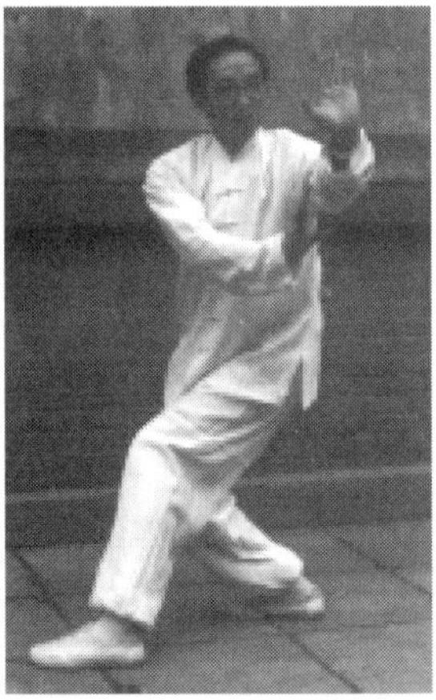

Figure 8-2

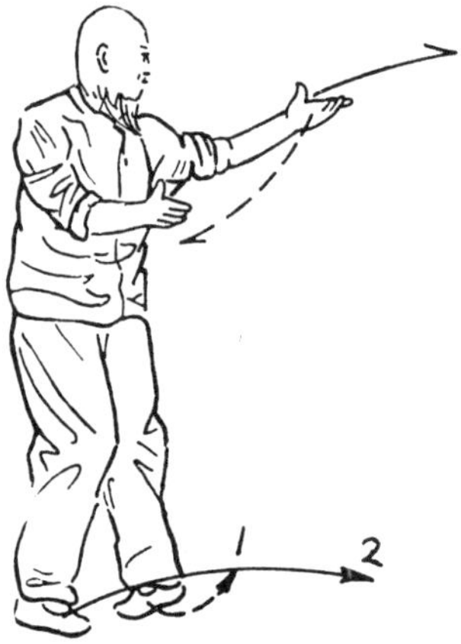

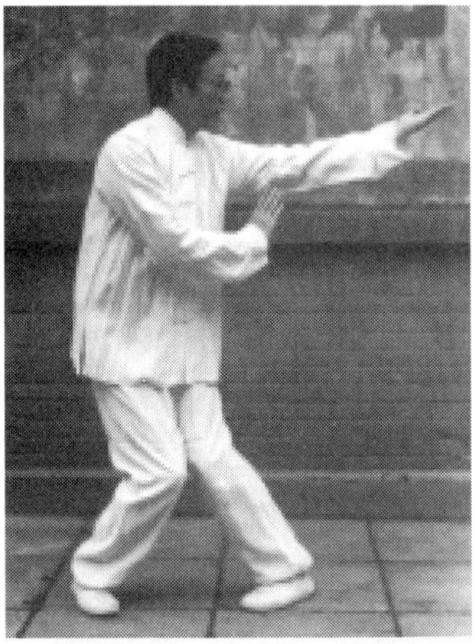

Figure 8-3

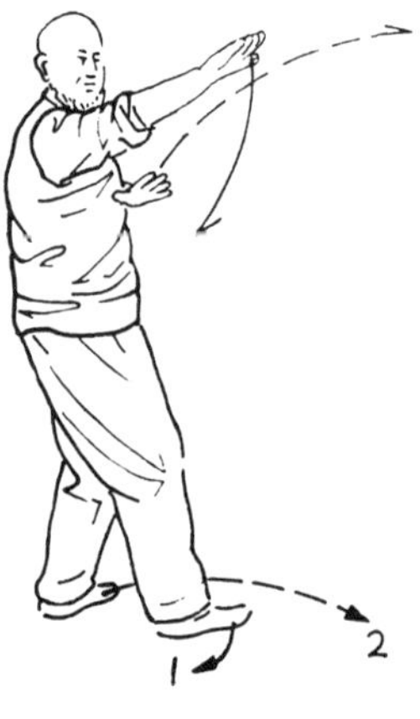

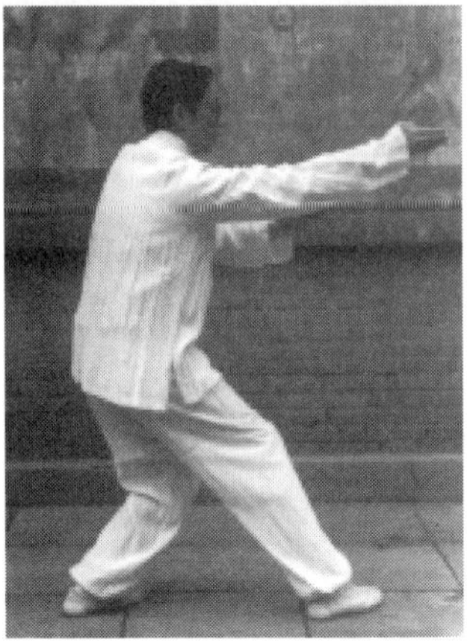

150

Exercises and Figures

Figure 8-4

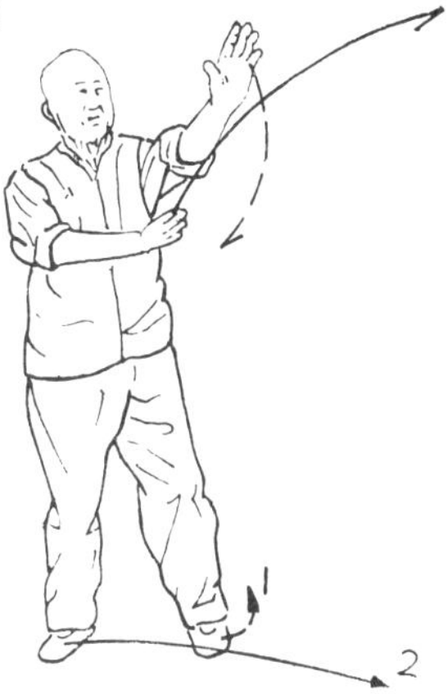

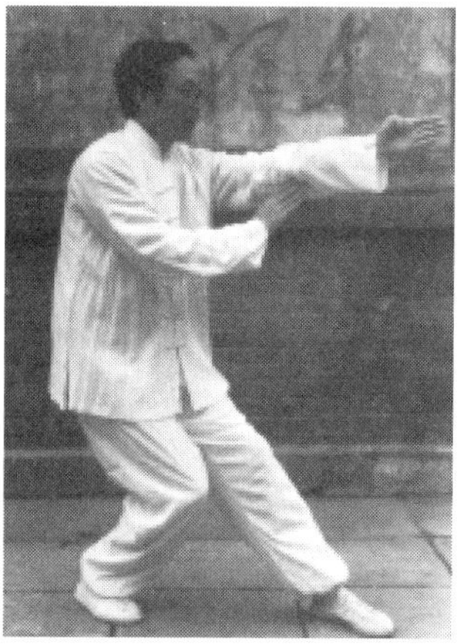

Figure 8-5

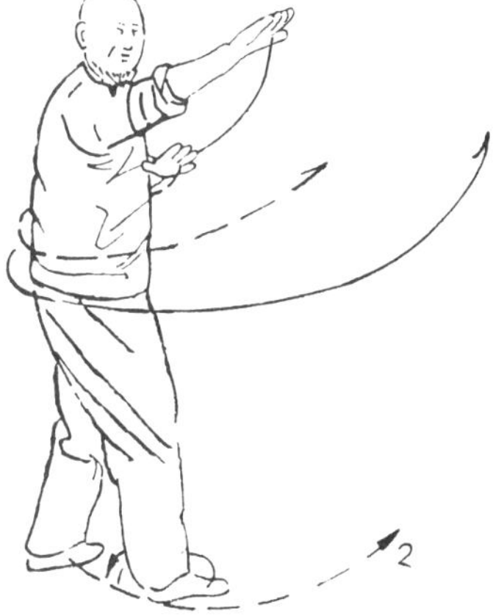

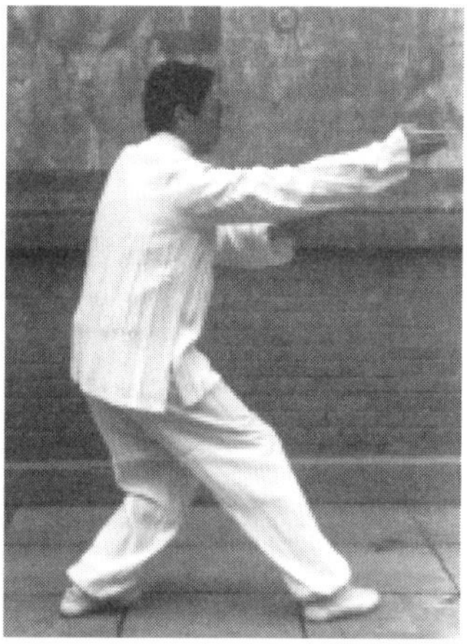

Figure 8-6

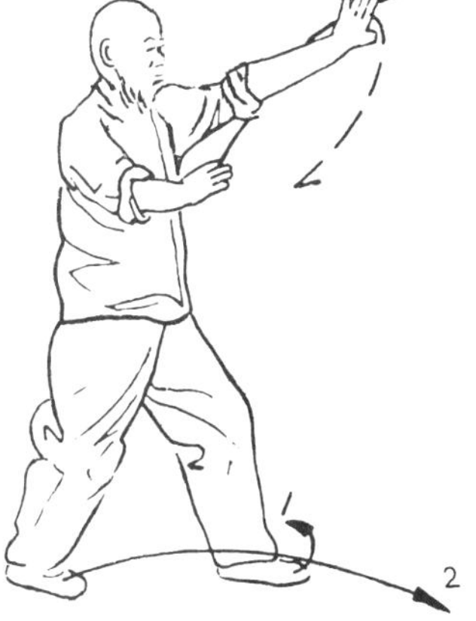

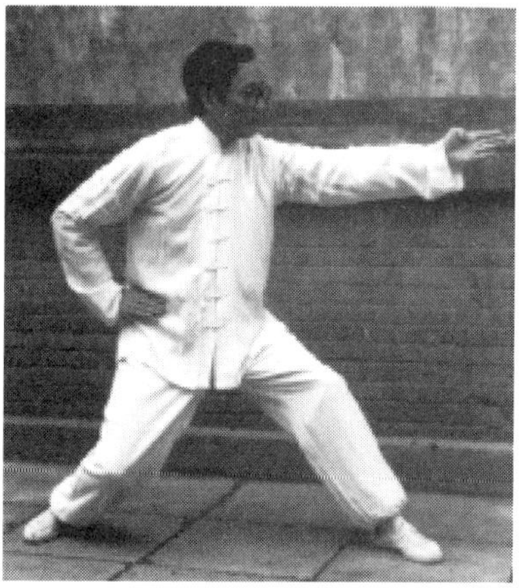

Liang Zhen Pu Eight Diagram Palm

Figure 8-7

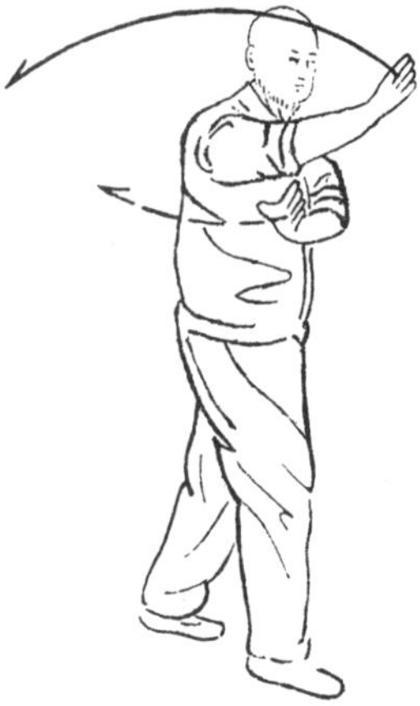

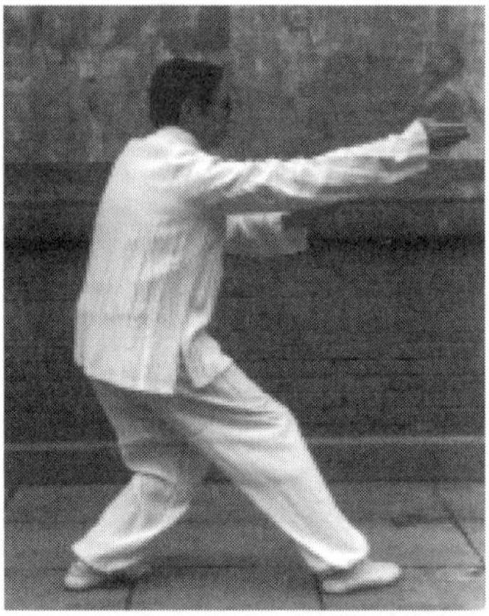

Figure 8-8

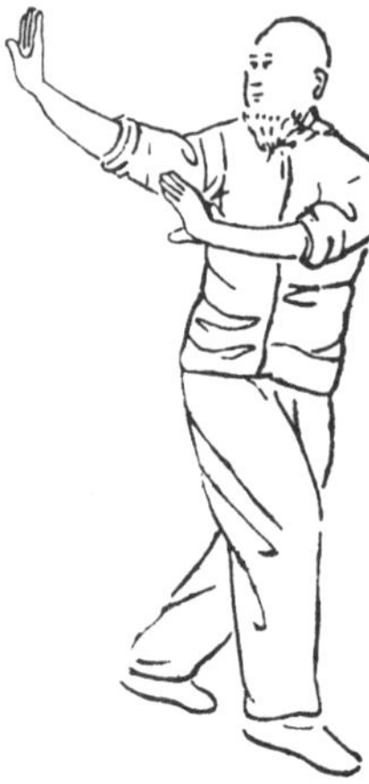

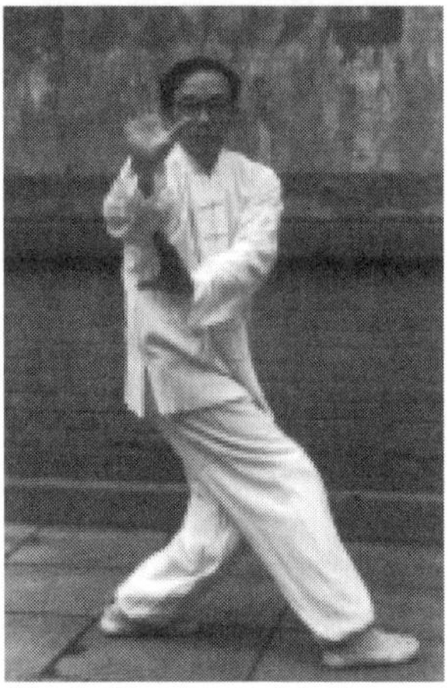

Exercises and Figures

EDITOR'S POSTSCRIPT

Master Li's treatise on Liang Zhen Pu's Ba Gua Zhang can be likened to a treasure sunken in the sands of a coral reef. With some effort, one stumbles upon jewels strewn about the ocean floor which only hint at the potential richness of the find. With persevering diligence, one can uncover beneath the sand much more than the already bountiful richness that has generously spread on the surface. While there are many details that could have been expounded upon in reference to the annotations, the time constraints imposed on us by the desire to release the first printing while Master Li was still with us (an effort nevertheless in vain due to his untimely passing on January 24, 1993), as well as keeping our focus on the original goal of presenting a faithful translation of this particular piece of work, compelled us to reserve such expansion for subsequent publication.

Those interested in pursuing these points in deeper and greater detail are encouraged to contact me in written correspondence and in person.

Note: Vincent Black is the designated representative for Li Zi Ming Ba Gua Zhang in North America and as such will assist interested parties in locating bona fide instructors of this lineage available for teaching. He can be contacted at: P.O. Box 36235, Tucson, Arizona 85740.

Liang Zhen Pu Eight Diagram Palm

About the Translator:

Huang Guo Qi

Mr. Huang Guo Qi was born on March 14, 1955 in Shanghai, China. From 1972 through 1977 he was a student in the Department of English Language and Literature at Fudan University in Shanghai, China. From 1980 to 1981 he was a graduate student in the Department of English Language at Jiaotong University in Shanghai, China.

Since 1977, Mr. Huang has been an instuctor at the Shanghai International Acupuncture Training Center affiliated with the Shanghai College of Traditional Chinese Medicine. He has over 15 years of experience translating books on traditional Chinese medicine and Chinese martial arts from the original Chinese to English.

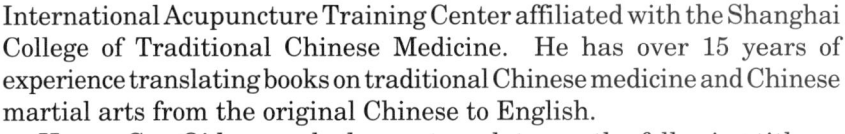

Huang Guo Qi has worked as co-translator on the following titles: *Chinese Acupuncture and Moxibustion* and *Essential Clinical Experience of Contemporary Chinese Famous Acupuncturists*

He was also the co-translator and co-editor of *State Standard - The Location of Acupoints*

Future titiles which Mr. Huang is currently translating include: *Dictionary of Acupuncture and Moxibustion*, *Acupuncture Treatment of 200 Commonly Encountered Diseases* and *Practical Clinical Compendium of Traditional Midicine: Volume Otorhinolaryngology*

Huang is the official coordinator and translator for the North American Tang Shou Tao Association in their endevors in mainland China and currently is working on several projects with the Association pertaining to martial arts and Chinese medicine.

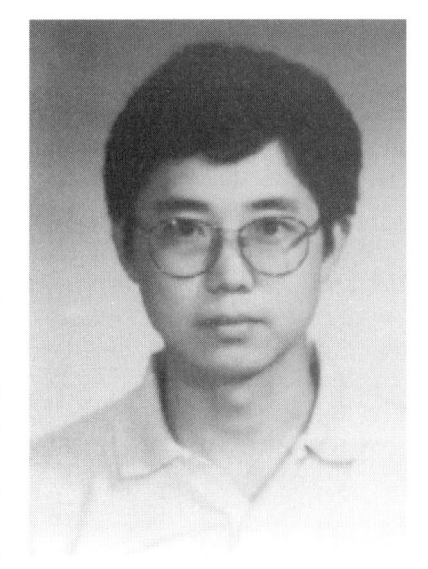